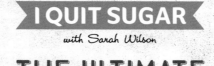

I QUIT SUGAR

with Sarah Wilson

THE ULTIMATE
CHOCOLATE
COOKBOOK

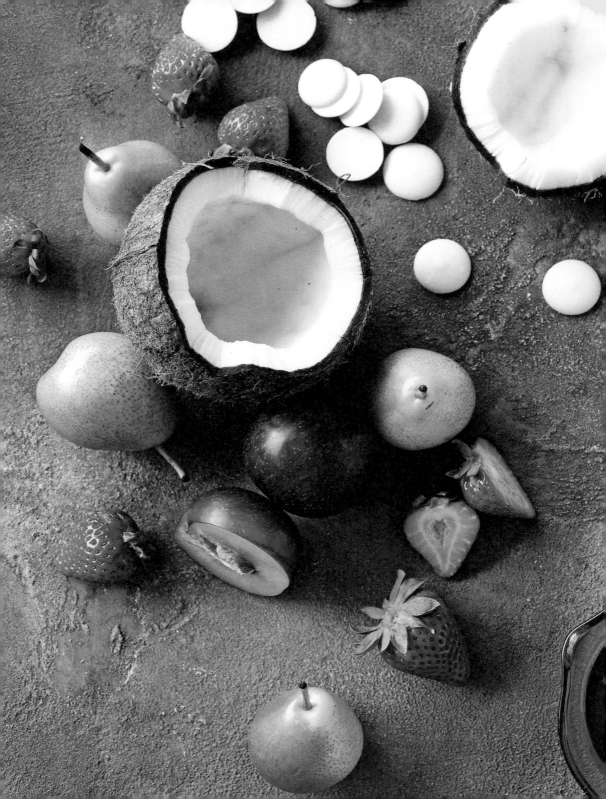

I QUIT SUGAR

with Sarah Wilson

THE ULTIMATE
CHOCOLATE
COOKBOOK

HEALTHY DESSERTS, KIDS'
TREATS AND GUILT-FREE
INDULGENCES

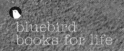

bluebird
books for life

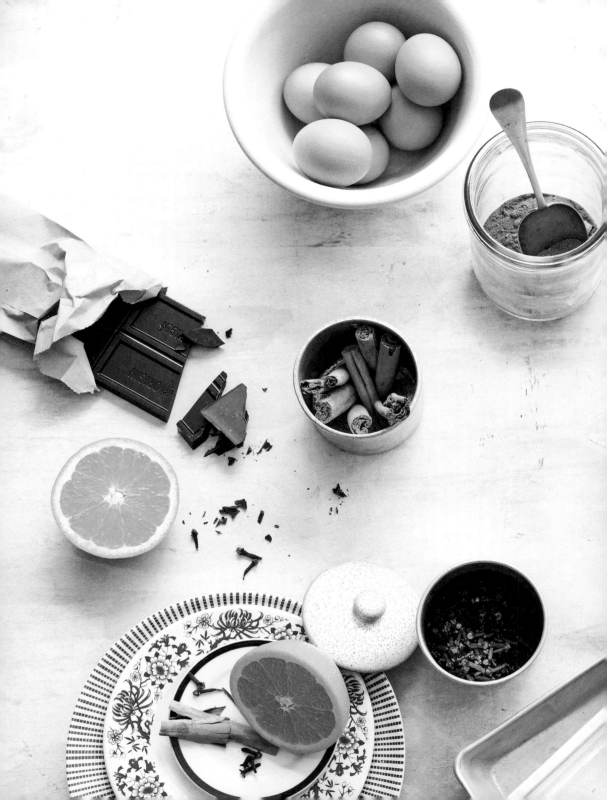

CONTENTS

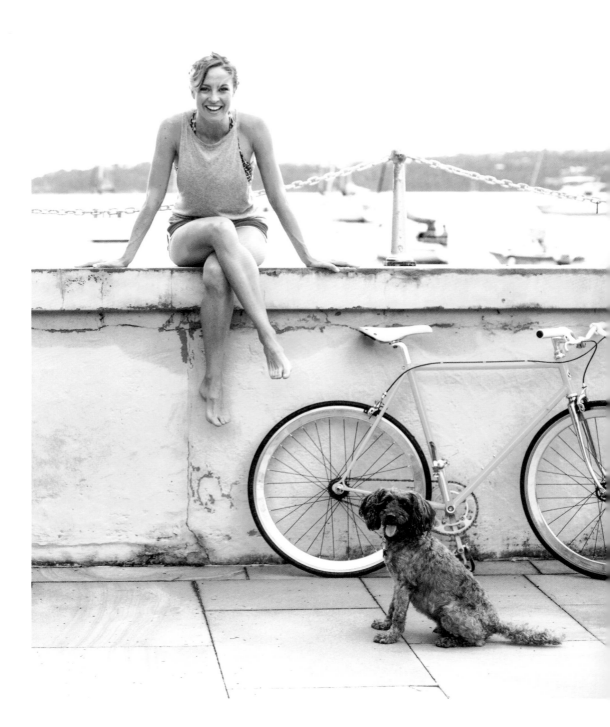

INTRODUCTION

This isn't our first chocolate cookbook. We have chocolate recipes coming out of our ears! But this is the first one that pulls all the best recipes into one single book. The 'ultimate' chocolate cookbook, if you like.

While it's true that you don't have to quit chocolate when you quit sugar, you do have to eat it correctly. Which for starters means not all the time. If you do want to eat it daily, aim for recipes that have only ½ teaspoon per serve. The rest are a 'sometimes' treat, to be savoured and enjoyed. To this end you'll notice that we put a big focus on portion control. Our recipes serve a crowd and are divvied up into rather small slices, bites and balls.

What else?

- Chocolate should always be made with raw cacao, not cocoa.
- When making your own raw chocolate, use virgin cold-pressed varieties of coconut oil.
- Start with less sweetener and add more if needed.
- Eat chocolate straight after a main meal to avoid it becoming a snack food.

Of course, the good thing about switching away from standard chocolate recipes to ours is that portion control is entirely possible. Our treats don't contain the highly addictive and bingey fructose and are made with lush, rich, nutrient-dense ingredients to ensure all the right appetite hormones are switched on when you bite in. And satiety can ensue!

To help you out, we've included a bunch of information that will tell you when a recipe is okay to eat daily, should be eaten mindfully or should be eaten rarely.

This new book also contains gluten-free, kid-friendly (nut-free), freezable and vegan options as well. Oh, and a whole bunch of fun quick fixes-for-one, some classic chocolatey treats pimped I Quit Sugar-style, and a lush sugar-free* Easter chapter…and …

In fact, I'm not sure why you're still reading. Time to jump into the recipes! Please do enjoy (mindfully) and feel free to share your results with me and the IQS Team on your social media using the hashtags #IQS and #IQSChocolate.

Much sated and nutrient-dense wellness to you,

Sarah
xx

*When we say sugar-free we mean fructose-free, because that's the stuff we're trying to avoid.

BEFORE WE START

Here's a little recap of all things chocolate.

Know the difference: caçao versus cocoa

Raw cacao powder: Made by cold-pressing unroasted cocoa beans. The process keeps the living enzymes in the cocoa and removes the fat (cacao butter).

Cocoa powder: Raw cacao that's been roasted at high temperatures. Sadly, roasting changes the molecular structure of the cocoa bean, reducing the enzyme content and lowering the overall nutritional value.

WE ADVISE USING RAW CACAO WHEREVER POSSIBLE.

However, standard cocoa powder can be substituted 1:1 if you're stuck or have an unfinished packet of the stuff in your store cupboard.

Cacao butter: The fat in cocoa beans that separates from the powder when the bean is cold-pressed (cacao) or roasted (cocoa).

Cacao liquor: Mostly referred to as 'cocoa mass', it's pure chocolate in liquid form. Made by pressing the whole cocoa bean and heating it at a very low temperature until it forms a paste, it is the main ingredient in most conventional chocolate.

Cacao nibs: Cocoa beans that have been separated from their husks and broken into small 'choc chip-like' chunks. Cacao nibs have higher antioxidant levels than blueberries, red wine and green tea. They also contain chromium, an important mineral for stabilising blood sugar and reducing appetite.

Carob: Some like to use carob as a substitute for chocolate. We wouldn't! It contains up to 50 per cent fructose. (The fructose content of cacao/cocoa is negligible.)

DID YOU KNOW?

The more cacao you add the stronger the flavour. If you're a dark chocolate fan, feel free to add a little extra, or to adjust the ratio of chocolate to other ingredients, in the various recipes.

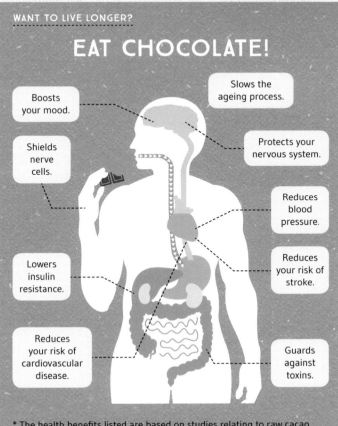

EAT CHOCOLATE!

Boosts your mood.

Slows the ageing process.

Shields nerve cells.

Protects your nervous system.

Reduces blood pressure.

Lowers insulin resistance.

Reduces your risk of stroke.

Reduces your risk of cardiovascular disease.

Guards against toxins.

* The health benefits listed are based on studies relating to raw cacao not store-bought, processed chocolate.

DID YOU KNOW?

Homemade chocolate can't go on picnics. Most of the homemade chocolate recipes from the cookbook use a combination of raw cacao butter, butter and coconut oil as a base, all of which have their own health benefits. All these ingredients are solid at cooler temperatures, but melt when left out (cacao butter at 35°C, butter at 30°C and coconut oil at 24°C). Which means, unless it's winter, or you live in Iceland, you need to eat it straight from the fridge or freezer.

THE DEAL WITH STORE-BOUGHT CHOCOLATE

In this cookbook some recipes invite you to use store-bought chocolate, in which case we advise using 85–90 per cent cocoa varieties. But we've kept these to a minimum; working with raw cacao is always best!

Dark chocolate can contain reasonably low amounts of sugar/fructose. Generally, whatever's not cocoa is sugar. So, a 70 per cent cocoa chocolate bar will contain about 30 per cent sugar. If you're eating a small 35 g bar, that's about 10.5 g sugar, or 2½ teaspoons. But bear in mind some 'dark chocolate' contains a meagre 30 per cent cocoa. We recommend you always turn the bar over to check the fine print!

> **DID YOU KNOW?**
>
> The darker the chocolate, the higher the cacao. And the higher the cacao, the more bitter it is. The flavanols are what make the chocolate bitter which is why the manufacturers often remove them – but it's those same flavanols that are responsible for many of chocolate's health benefits.

STORE-BOUGHT CHOCOLATE: WHAT TO LOOK FOR

Choose those containing:

✓ **85 per cent cocoa:** This stuff is okay to use sparingly in your cooking, or to eat a few squares at a time. A 100 g block will contain 15 g sugar.

✓ **99 per cent cocoa:** Hard to source and very intense in flavour.

✓ **Stevia:** Read up on stevia on page 6. Beware: those chocolates with stevia often also contain other sweeteners as well. Don't be fooled by the 'stevia sweetened' labelling. Look closer.

✓ **Glucose:** This is not a licence to go crazy on glucose. Even non-fructose sugars, such as glucose, are not good to eat in large quantities and will cause insulin wobbliness too, albeit in a far more manageable way.

✓ **Rice malt syrup:** Read up on rice malt syrup on page 6.

✓ **4g sugar or less per 100 g:** This is a basic rule we stick to when eating all packaged foods.

✓ **Organic:** Where possible we recommend organic brands. This ensures there's less rubbish being added to your chocolate and, in our experience, these brands have a bit more environmental awareness than some others.

Avoid those containing:

✕ **Agave:** Contains 60–90 per cent fructose.

✕ **Aspartame:** A chemical sweetener linked to the formation of cancer cells.

✕ **Coconut nectar:** Contains 38–50 per cent fructose.

✕ **Coconut sugar:** Contains 38–50 per cent fructose.

✕ **Honey:** Contains 38 per cent fructose.

✕ **Palm oil (PGPR):** Most commercial chocolates contain unhealthy poly-unsaturated oils, often palm oil, or PGPR. These oils cause a lot of oxidative stress in our body and are linked to cancer and heart disease. Palm oil also comes with a host of ethical issues.

We also recommend avoiding these sweeteners:

✕ Fruit concentrate	✕ Corn syrup	✕ GMO ingredients
✕ Fruit purée	✕ High Fructose Corn Syrup (HFCS)	✕ Polydextrose
✕ Maple syrup	✕ Inulin	✕ Soy lecithin
✕ Fructans	✕ Maltitol	✕ Sugar alcohols
✕ Cane sugar	✕ Vegetable oil	✕ Skimmed milk solids
✕ Golden syrup	✕ Canola/rapeseed oil	✕ Barley malt extract
✕ Molasses	✕ Sucrose	✕ Maltose
✕ Dates	✕ Sorbitol	✕ Invert sugar
✕ Maple sugar		✕ Isomalt

Your call:

→ **Xylitol:** Xylitol is one of two safe sugar alcohols. Our livers eventually convert xylitol to glucose, so it ultimately has no ill effect on humans.

→ **Erythritol:** Another sugar alcohol used to cut through stevia. There's no conclusive evidence on it but we find it can make your tummy grumbly.

→ **Monk fruit extract:** Again, this is used to sweeten foods but lack of solid science means we choose to stay away from the stuff.

→ **Saccharin:** Not approved in other Western countries.

→ **Cyclamate:** Not approved in other Western countries.

→ **Alitame:** Not approved in other Western countries.

→ **Dextrose:** Dextrose is pure glucose, containing no fructose, so your body will detect it and process it. However, you'll need a large amount to sweeten food so we tend to avoid it as much as possible.

THE SWEETENERS

More about the good stuff.

Rice malt syrup: This is a blend of maltose and glucose made from fermented, cooked rice. You can use this in place of sugar or honey in recipes, roughly in a 1:1 ratio. Some folk say it is less sweet than honey and sugar. We beg to differ and tend to put less of it in our recipes than many others would. You can find it in health food shops and many supermarkets (in the baking section) and it costs about the same as honey. Look for brands that list organic rice as the only ingredient.

Stevia: This is a natural sweetener, derived from a leaf similar to mint and is composed of stevioside (which is 300 times sweeter than sugar) and rebaudioside (450 times sweeter than sugar). Stevia comes as a liquid or mixed with erythritol to form a granule and the latter version is readily available in many supermarkets (in the baking section).

When we refer to stevia in this book, we mean the granulated form. Most stevia granules can be used as you would sugar, although we tend to use about a third less.

If you're using the liquid form, keep in mind these conversions:

- 1 cup (200 g) sugar/granulated stevia = 1 teaspoon liquid stevia.
- 1 tablespoon sugar/granulated stevia = 6–9 drops liquid stevia.
- 1 teaspoon sugar/granulated stevia = 2–4 drops liquid stevia.

Another thing to keep in mind: Stevia can be bitter if used in excess so we tend to recommend rice malt syrup for kids.

Other sweeteners that are okay to use in moderation are xylitol and erythritol (sugar alcohols that can be digested by our bodies) and dextrose (100 per cent glucose). However, we tend to avoid both. Rice malt syrup is best as it breaks down as a complex carbohydrate thus releasing glucose into the body slowly. Also stay clear of natural fructose like coconut nectar and agave. Both are equally as potent in their forms and will cause insulin spikes, which is what we're trying to avoid.

The rest: Don't touch, most have been shown to be either potentially carcinogenic or entirely indigestible, and could cause myriad health issues. Many of the fake sugars available are banned in parts of Europe, deemed unsafe. 'Nuff said.

HOW TO MELT CHOCOLATE

A number of recipes call for you to melt down store-bought chocolate. To do so, you need to know a few things:

1. Chocolate's melting point is low, which makes it very easy to burn.

2. If heated above 95°C over an open flame, it will scorch.
   This damages the good oils and wakes up the harmful compounds.

Some tips

CHOP IT UNIFORMLY. Don't try to melt a whole bar or block.

USE A DOUBLE BOILER. Or a bain marie if you have one, or simply place a metal bowl – ceramic can work too – over a small saucepan with 2 cm of water in it. (Avoid all contact with water. Otherwise it will 'seize'.) Simmer gently, stirring the chocolate/cacao butter until melted. Take it slowly and gently!

USE A RUBBER SPATULA. Never use a wooden spoon as it absorbs liquid from the chocolate and never use a metal spoon as it conducts heat, causing the chocolate to overheat.

STIR. Chocolate retains its shape when melted, so the only way to know if it is actually melted is to stir it. Stir continuously until your chocolate is shiny, smooth and completely melted.

GO SLOW AND LOW. When chocolate is overheated, it becomes lumpy or grainy. Melt slowly over very low heat. Did we mention slow?

CHOCOLATE WILL MELT FASTER THAN OTHER LIQUIDS. If you're melting it with milk, cream or coconut cream, melt the other liquids first. (This also helps prevent the chocolate from seizing if it's melted with cold liquids.)

MY CHOCOLATE HAS SEIZED! CAN I FIX IT?

If your melted chocolate has turned into a lumpy mess, don't toss it! While it can't be used for silky sauces, it can still be used for baking. Stir solid coconut oil into the chocolate, using 1 tablespoon for every 150 g of chocolate. Stir gently and evenly until the chocolate has loosened and the oil is incorporated. Add this mixture to baked goods like brownies and cakes where chocolate is called for.

HOW MUCH CHOCOLATE IS TOO MUCH?

We've said it already, but we'd like to highlight again that most of the recipes in this cookbook are treats, to be consumed as just that. Apart from the breakfast chapter, they're not 'every day' foods.

So, while they contain little or no fructose, quite a number contain glucose (in the form of rice malt syrup), which, while able to be metabolised by our bodies (unlike fructose), still causes insulin spikes. Remember, whenever we say 'sugar-free' we mean 'fructose-free'.

Most recipes in this book (okay, all!) are sweet in flavour, which may continue to drive the very same sweet addiction we are trying to rid ourselves of. Each time we consume something sweet, whether it contains fructose, glucose or artificial sweeteners, our brain registers this fact and primes our body (with hormones and chemicals) to deal with them. In general, though, feel confident that most of the treats in this book are not addictive and contain plenty of healthy fats, which will satiate you and trigger the 'I'm full' switch in your brain, ensuring you won't binge on them. In other words: unlike when you eat commercial, sugar-laden chocolate, your body will tell you when you've had enough of the chocolate in this book.

THING TO KNOW?

We're not big on waste! The idea of you heading out to buy a jar of something that you use once, and then have it sit at the back of your fridge for months before being tossed, makes us sad. So how about this: buy an ingredient or two at a time and cook a bunch of recipes that make use of them. Then move on to the next exotic ingredient.

A STORE-CUPBOARD GUIDE

These are a bunch of common ingredients you'll come across in this book. Some might be unfamiliar to you, so we're highlighting a few things to look for when buying them.

Cacao butter

Comes in big chunks and needs to be grated and melted down before using. You can also sometimes buy it as 'buttons'. It tends to be a little pricey and hard to find (best to buy it online), which is why some prefer to use butter or coconut oil instead. However, it does make for a creamier, 'fullness of mouth' chocolate that doesn't melt as readily.

Look for: Brands that are cold-pressed rather than heated, as heating may destroy the vitamin E content.

Chia seeds

A native South American seed, rich in omega-3 fatty acids, protein, fibre, calcium, magnesium, potassium and vitamin C. These are great to add to chocolate treats for a choc chip-like crunch and to transform an indulgence into a protein-packed meal.

Look for: 100 per cent natural (GMO, preservative free), sustainably farmed, organic or fair trade seeds. Try white versions to mix things up a little! For our Bluffer's Guide to Chia Seeds, visit us at IQuitSugar.com.

Coconut butter

This is basically whole coconut flesh puréed into a spread that tastes oddly like white chocolate. You can buy it in many health food shops (it's pricey) or make your own (see page 156).

Look for: Unsweetened brands that only use 100 per cent raw coconut. Steer clear of flavoured coconut butters, such as 'cacao coconut butter' as these are often sweetened with agave.

Coconut oil

A wonderfully sweet oil extracted from the kernel or meat of mature coconuts and easy to buy in health food shops, online and in many supermarkets. You can catch up on why it's so healthy on our website. But for present purposes, it's fantastic for making simple chocolates – the oil is sweet enough not to require much (if any) additional sweetener.

Look for: Wild harvested varieties that have been transported in cold storage containers. Also brands that clearly state they're 100 per cent organic, raw and virgin.

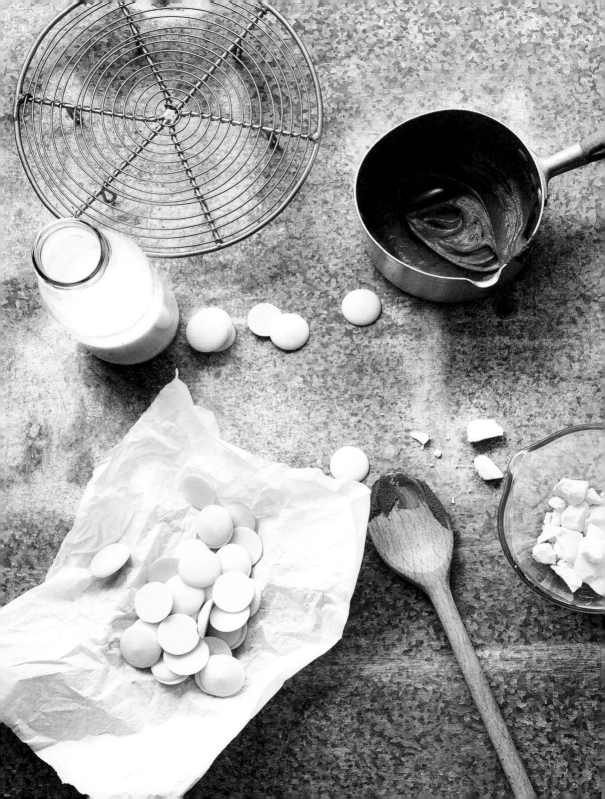

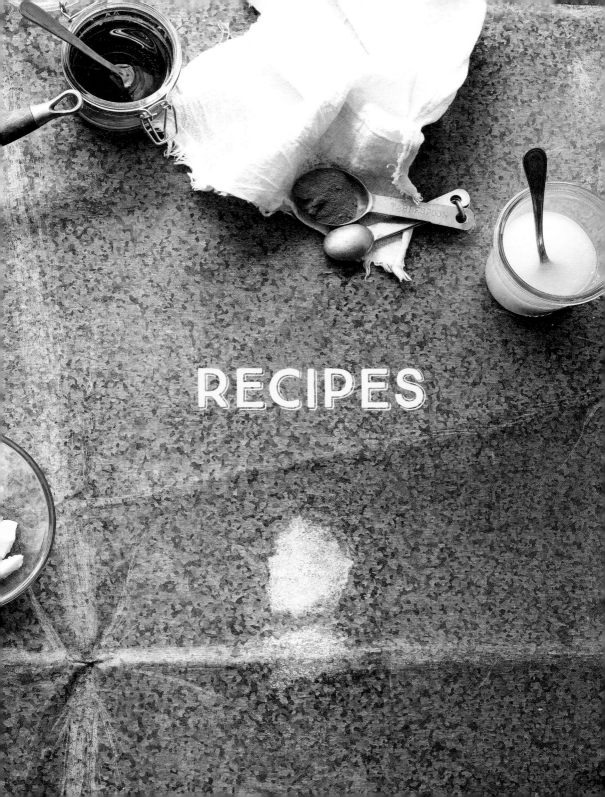

RECIPES

HOW TO USE THIS BOOK

We're almost there!

Just a few handy instructions on how to navigate this book and then you'll be ready to cook.

1. Use the Store-Cupboard Guide (see page 9) to find out what you can make with a particular ingredient.

2. Make some substitutions:

> RAW CACAO POWDER = COCOA POWDER.
>
> NUT FLOURS = ANY PLAIN FLOUR,
> BUT ADD A LITTLE EXTRA OIL/BUTTER.
>
> COCONUT FLAKES = SHREDDED COCONUT = DESICCATED COCONUT.
> A word of caution though: many desiccated brands are sweetened,
> so check yours!

3. Look out for these icons:

P **Paleo:** Recipes that are grain-, dairy-, sugar- and legume-free.

GF **Gluten-free:** Recipes that don't contain gluten.

DF **Dairy-free:** Recipes that don't contain dairy or dairy products.

V **Vegan:** Recipes with no animal products. Many of the recipes that do contain butter can be altered to include coconut oil instead.

❄ **Freeze:** Recipes that require storage in the freezer, or can be frozen for a later date.

KF **Kid-friendly:** Recipes that contain zero nuts and/or are ideal as a treat for the kids.

Now, let's make some chocolate!

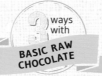

3 ways with

BASIC RAW CHOCOLATE

We suggest experimenting to see what version you like (playing with the different sweeteners, too). You'll see these recipes scattered throughout the book. But first, a few things to note:

- Working with cacao butter takes a little more work (shaving and melting) and the stuff is expensive. But it does produce a creamier result and doesn't melt as easily as the coconut oil versions.

- Working with coconut oil is simple and we find you don't need as much sweetener (take out a little from the recipes if you like), but it doesn't seem to 'grab' the cacao as well as the cacao butter does. Plus it must be eaten quickly from the fridge/freezer (it melts if the temperature is anything over about 24°C).

- You can keep a batch in the fridge or freezer for several weeks and remelt as required.

BASIC RAW CHOCOLATE #1
(WITH CACAO BUTTER)

GF V P ❄

MAKES 1⅓ cups
(320 ml)

COOKING TIME
5 minutes

1 cup (225 g) raw cacao butter, buttons or shavings

⅓ cup (30 g) raw cacao powder

1–2 teaspoons granulated stevia or 1–2 tablespoons rice malt syrup

2 pinches of sea salt

1. Melt the cacao butter gently, stirring until dissolved. Blend/mix with the rest of the ingredients until smooth/combined.

BASIC RAW CHOCOLATE #2

(WITH A BLEND OF CACAO BUTTER + COCONUT OIL)

MAKES 1⅓ cups
(320 ml)

COOKING TIME
5 minutes

½ cup (115 g) raw cacao
butter, buttons or shavings

½ cup (115 g) coconut oil,
softened

⅓ cup (30 g) raw cacao
powder

1–2 teaspoons granulated
stevia or 1–2 tablespoons
rice malt syrup

2 pinches of sea salt

1. Melt the cacao butter gently, stirring until dissolved.
    Blend/mix with the rest of the ingredients until
    smooth/combined.

BASIC RAW CHOCOLATE #3

(WITH COCONUT OIL)

MAKES 1⅓ cups
(320 ml)

COOKING TIME
5 minutes

1 cup (225 g) coconut oil,
softened

⅓ cup (30 g) raw cacao
powder

2 pinches of sea salt

1–2 teaspoons granulated
stevia or 1–2 tablespoons
rice malt syrup

1. Blend all ingredients until combined.

BREAKFAST SPECIALS

Chocolate for breakfast? Yep! These recipes are all protein rich and packed with mood-boosting cacao – just what you need to start your day right.

CHOCOLATEY
PANCAKE STACK

These pancakes are super simple, fluffy and packed with protein.
Did we mention they're chocolate? What more could you want?!

MAKES 6

PREPARATION TIME
5 minutes

COOKING TIME
10 minutes

2 eggs

1 tablespoon rice malt syrup

1 teaspoon vanilla extract

¾ cup (175 ml) almond milk (or milk of your choice)

2 cups (200 g) almond meal

pinch of sea salt

2 tablespoons raw cacao powder

1 teaspoon ground cinnamon

1 teaspoon baking powder

coconut oil, butter or ghee, for greasing

berries and Basic Raw Chocolate (see page 13), to serve

1. Whisk together the eggs, rice malt syrup, vanilla and milk.

2. Add in the almond meal, salt, cacao, cinnamon and baking powder and mix until smooth.

3. Melt some coconut oil, butter or ghee in a large pan on medium heat. Add 4 tablespoons of the pancake mixture into the pan. Cook until the sides of the pancake are firm and a few bubbles escape from the top, about 3 minutes.

4. Carefully flip the pancake and cook for another 45 seconds. Remove from the heat and repeat with remaining mixture. Serve topped with berries and raw chocolate.

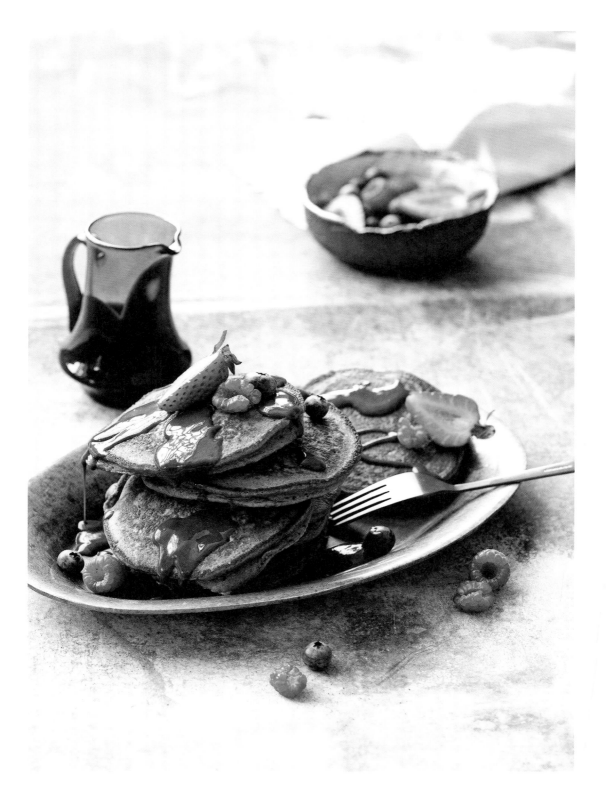

NOURISHING CACAO
SMOOTHIE BOWL

Use a spoon to slurp up your smoothie and enjoy the delightful caramel flavour of the cashews and banana throughout. By the way, this will keep you going until lunchtime!

SERVES 2

PREPARATION TIME

5 minutes

⅓ cup (40 g) pre-soaked cashews

1 banana, chopped and frozen

2 teaspoons chia seeds

1 cup (250 ml) natural full-fat yoghurt

1 cup (250 ml) almond milk (or milk of your choice)

2 tablespoons raw cacao powder

3 drops liquid stevia, optional

1 teaspoon maca powder, optional

coconut flakes, to serve

1. Throw all the ingredients into a blender and blend until smooth.

2. Pour into two bowls and allow to sit for 5 minutes in the fridge. Top with the coconut flakes, to serve.

BREAKFAST BERRY 'N' CHOC WHIP

This berry whip tastes like dessert in a glass! To make it nut-free and a great option for kids, use dairy or coconut milk in place of almond milk and omit LSA.

SERVES 2

PREPARATION TIME
2 minutes

1 cup (150 g) frozen mixed berries

1½ cups (370 ml) almond milk (or milk of your choice)

1½ tablespoons raw cacao powder

1 teaspoon coconut oil

1 tablespoon flaxseeds or LSA (linseed, sunflower seed and almond blend), optional

2–3 drops liquid stevia, optional (or ¼ frozen banana)

1. Combine all the ingredients in a blender and blend until smooth. Serve.

CACAO AND SWEET POTATO WAFFLES

Dig out your dusty waffle makers – they're making a comeback! We've put a healthy spin on an old favourite by adding some naturally sweet spices and some vitamin-rich sweet potato. Yum!

MAKES 2

PREPARATION TIME
5 minutes

COOKING TIME
5 minutes

coconut oil, butter or ghee, for greasing

1 cup (100 g) almond meal

⅓ cup (75 ml) coconut milk

2 eggs, whisked

2 tablespoons raw cacao powder

1 tablespoon rice malt syrup

1 teaspoon ground cinnamon

1 teaspoon vanilla powder or extract, optional

1 teaspoon baking powder

½ cup (60 g) grated sweet potato

pinch of sea salt

butter, to serve (we prefer peanut butter!)

1. Preheat your waffle iron and grease (if necessary).

2. Combine all of the ingredients in a large bowl.

3. Pour approximately half the mixture onto your waffle iron and cook for roughly 3 minutes or until cooked through. Repeat with the remaining mixture. Serve with butter.

> **TRICKY TIP**
>
> Make up a batch of waffles and freeze. Simply take one straight from the freezer and toast for an instant snack or quick breakfast option.

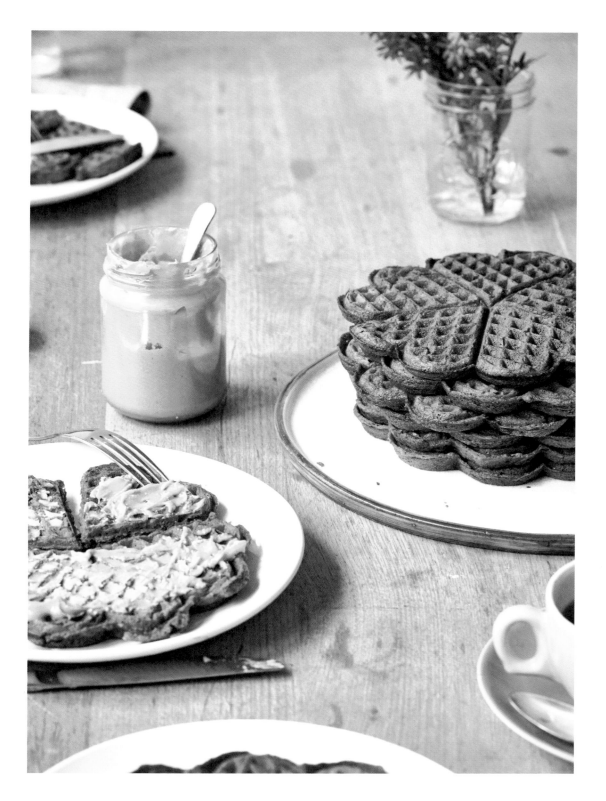

KALE 'N' CACAO BIRCHER

The beauty of this bircher is the sneaky injection of greens. Make up a batch the night before and you'll have a complete meal with minimum effort.

SERVES 2

PREPARATION TIME

10 minutes +
overnight

4 tablespoons nuts of your choice

2 tablespoons shredded coconut

1 teaspoon chia seeds

1 tablespoon flaxseeds or LSA (linseed, sunflower seed and almond blend)

4 kale leaves, destalked

1 tablespoon vanilla protein powder, optional (omit for paleo)

1½ tablespoons raw cacao powder

1 teaspoon ground cinnamon

1 teaspoon maca powder, optional

½ cup (50 g) oats or ½ cup (85 g) buckwheat groats

pinch of granulated stevia, optional

1 cup (250 ml) almond milk (or milk of your choice)

fresh or frozen berries and natural full-fat yoghurt, to serve

1. In a blender or food processor combine the nuts, coconut, chia seeds, flaxseeds/LSA, kale, protein powder, cacao, cinnamon and maca.

2. Stir oats/buckwheat groats and milk through the mixture. Spoon mixture into two jars, cover and sit in the fridge overnight. To serve, top with berries and yoghurt.

AUTUMN-SPICED BREAKFAST BROWNIES

A change in season often inspires us to change the ingredients we cook with. Ground yourself and warm from the inside out with this chocolatey brownie, loaded with autumnal spices and sweet pumpkin.

SERVES 4

PREPARATION TIME
10 minutes

COOKING TIME
25 minutes

1 cup (250 ml) Pumpkin Purée (see page 166)

¼ cup (50 g) almond butter

½ cup (50 g) almond meal

1 tablespoon rice malt syrup

¼ cup (25 g) raw cacao powder

2 eggs, whisked

1 teaspoon ground cinnamon

½ teaspoon ground nutmeg

½ teaspoon ground ginger

1 teaspoon vanilla powder or extract, optional

½ teaspoon sea salt

1 teaspoon baking powder

coconut cream or natural full-fat yoghurt, to serve

1. Preheat oven to 180°C (gas 4) and line a 22 cm square brownie tin.

2. Combine all of the ingredients in a medium bowl, and mix well until a smooth batter forms.

3. Transfer the batter to the lined tin, and bake for 20–25 minutes, or until the edges are just firm to the touch. You want it to be quite soft and pudding-like in the middle.

4. Allow to cool in the tin, then scoop into bowls and serve with cream or yoghurt.

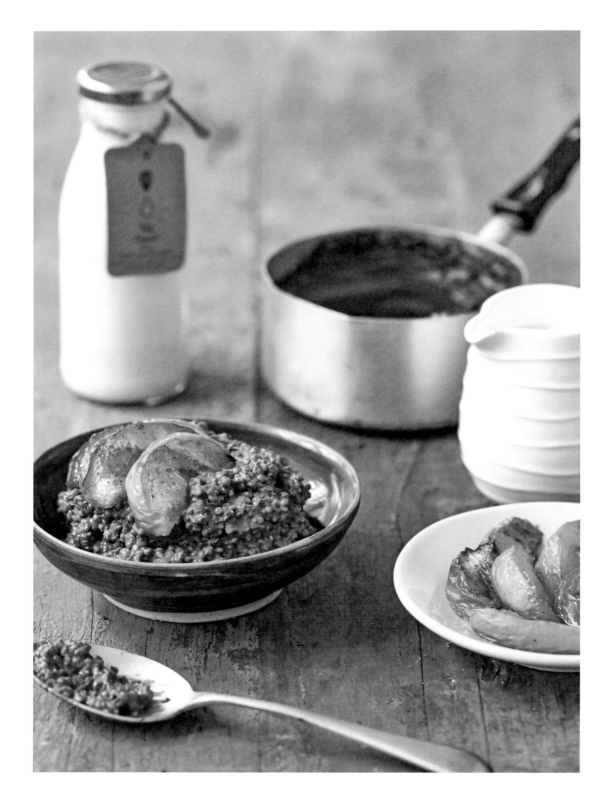

SWEET CHOCOLATE RISOTTO WITH CINNAMON GRILLED PEACHES

Enjoy this rich, warming dish in the cooler months and experience a boost in mood and energy.

SERVES 4

PREPARATION TIME
5 minutes

COOKING TIME
20 minutes

1 cup (170 g) dried quinoa, thoroughly rinsed

1 litre almond milk (or milk of your choice)

1½ tablespoons rice malt syrup or 6 drops of liquid stevia

2 teaspoons vanilla powder or extract

¼ cup (25 g) raw cacao powder

2 peaches, cored and sliced into segments

2 teaspoons coconut oil, melted

2 teaspoons ground cinnamon

½ cup (120 ml) coconut milk or cream to serve, optional

1. Place quinoa, milk, rice malt syrup, vanilla and cacao in a medium saucepan and stir. Bring quinoa and liquid to the boil and then reduce heat to a low simmer. Cook quinoa until tender and 95 per cent of the liquid has been absorbed and the quinoa has sprouted 'tails'. Remove from heat and stir.

2. Meanwhile coat peaches with coconut oil and sprinkle with cinnamon. Place peaches on a lined baking tray under the grill. Cook until golden and caramelised (about 7 minutes).

3. Pour cooked quinoa into four bowls, drizzle with coconut milk/cream and top with grilled peaches.

CHOCOLATE COURGETTE LOAF

MAKES 1 loaf

PREPARATION TIME
20 minutes

COOKING TIME
45 minutes

coconut oil, butter or ghee,
for greasing

2 cups (450 g) courgette, grated,
drained in a sieve

¾ cup (175 g) unsalted butter,
softened

⅓ cup (75 ml) rice malt syrup

2 eggs

2½ cups (300 g) gluten-free flour

½ cup (50 g) raw cacao powder

2 teaspoons bicarbonate of soda

½ teaspoon vanilla powder

½ teaspoon salt

1 teaspoon ground cinnamon

cacao nibs and chia seeds,
to serve

1. Preheat oven to 180°C (gas 4). Grease a 22 cm x 13 cm loaf tin. Place grated courgette in a sieve or colander and sprinkle with a pinch of salt. Allow to sit for 5 minutes then squeeze excess water out.

2. Melt butter and rice malt syrup on medium heat. Allow to cool for 5 minutes.

3. Combine eggs with butter/syrup mixture.

4. Thoroughly mix together flour, cacao, bicarbonate of soda, vanilla, salt and cinnamon in a large bowl until combined.

5. Combine the wet mixture with the grated courgette. Slowly add the dry ingredients to the wet.

6. Pour mixture into greased loaf tin and smooth out top. Sprinkle cacao nibs and chia seeds on top if desired.

7. Bake in the oven for 35–40 minutes, or until a skewer inserted into the centre comes out clean. Remove from the oven and allow to cool for 5 minutes before transferring out of the tin to a wire rack.

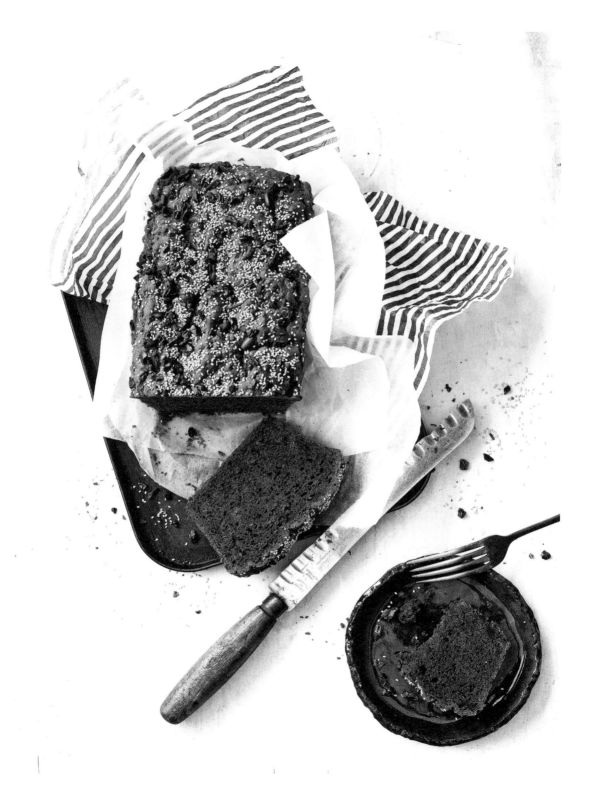

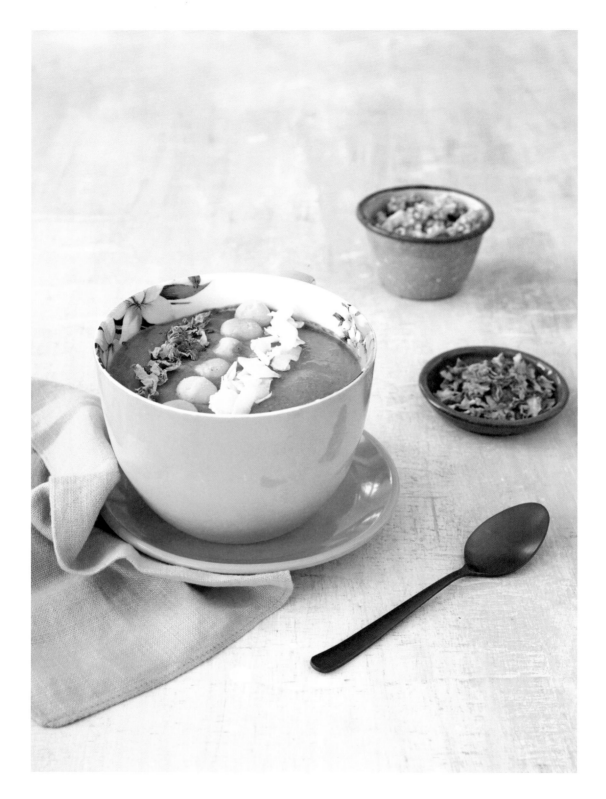

CHOCO-MACADAMIA
CRUNCH SMOOTHIE BOWL

This chocolate smoothie has it all: spinach for a good dose of greens, chia seeds
for some good fats and raw cacao powder for an antioxidant boost!

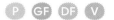

SERVES 2

PREPARATION TIME
7 minutes

3 cups (750 ml) almond milk

¼ cup (40 g) chia seeds

1 banana, chopped and frozen

⅔ cup (80 g) macadamias, soaked in
water for 4 hours or overnight
+ extra for serving

¼ cup (25 g) raw cacao powder

1 cup (50 g) baby spinach leaves

8 frozen coconut cream cubes

1 teaspoon ground cinnamon

2 teaspoons coconut flakes,
to serve

1 teaspoon edible flowers,
to serve

1. Throw all ingredients (except the coconut flakes, extra macadamias and
    edible flowers) into a blender and blend until smooth.

2. Pour into two small bowls and allow to sit for 5 minutes in the fridge,
    this will allow the chia seeds to plump up and thicken.

3. After chilling, remove from the fridge and top each bowl with
    macadamias, coconut flakes and edible flowers to serve.

TRICKY TIP

Coconut cream cubes are super easy to make. Just pour a tin of coconut
cream into your ice cube tray and freeze until set. Adding these to your
smoothie bowl gives them a great eat-with-a-spoon consistency.

CHOCOLATE GRANOLA CLUSTERS

This is a mish-mash version of Sarah's original Coco-Nutty Granola in her first cookbook. It adds a good dose of raw cacao powder for a chocolatey hit!

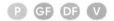

SERVES 2

PREPARATION TIME
5 minutes

COOKING TIME
20 minutes

3 cups (175 g) coconut flakes

2 cups (250 g) mixed nuts and seeds, roughly chopped

2 tablespoons chia seeds

1 teaspoon ground cinnamon, optional

¼ cup (50 g) coconut oil, melted

1 tablespoon rice malt syrup

½ cup (50 g) raw cacao powder

2 tablespoons cacao nibs

1. Preheat the oven to 120°C (gas ½) and line a baking tray with baking paper.

2. Combine all the ingredients in a large mixing bowl, then spread evenly on the tray. Bake for 15–20 minutes until golden, turning halfway through the cooking time.

3. Once nicely browned, remove from the oven and allow to cool. Place into containers or tightly sealed jars and store for up to two weeks.

> **TRICKY TIP**
>
> Serve ¾ cup (65 g) of Chocolate Granola Clusters with a large dollop of yoghurt for a delicious and filling breakfast.

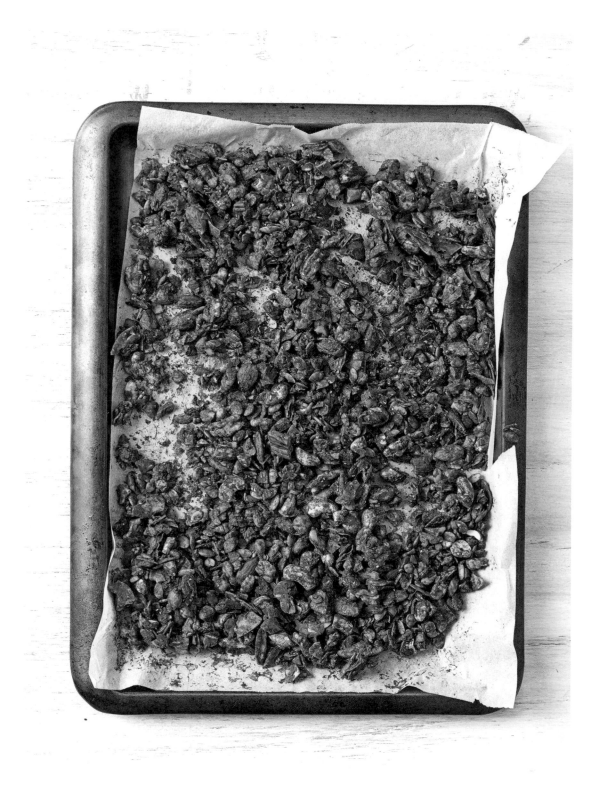

FRIED EGGS WITH MOLE SAUCE

Now, bear with us. Eggs and chocolate does sound weird but if you get the balance of this traditional mole right you'll delight your tastebuds with a new flavour combination and a nutrient-packed breakfast.

SERVES 2

PREPARATION TIME
10 minutes

COOKING TIME
10 minutes

4 eggs

2 teaspoons coconut oil

2 slices gluten-free bread or sourdough, optional

MOLE SAUCE

3 tablespoons raw cacao powder

1 tablespoon pumpkin seeds

1 tablespoon sesame seeds

½ tablespoon dried oregano

1 teaspoon ground cumin

pinch of sea salt, to taste

⅓ cup (15 g) fresh coriander, roughly chopped

1 tablespoon rice malt syrup

½ x 400 g can chopped tomatoes

2 teaspoons dried chilli flakes

1 tablespoon nut butter

1. Combine all of the mole ingredients in a food processor and blitz until completely smooth.

2. Heat a medium pan with coconut oil. Pour mole mixture into pan and cook for 5–10 minutes until sauce is reduced and fragrant. Add water if the mixture is too thick.

3. Set mixture aside. Fry eggs in coconut oil and toast up some bread. Serve eggs with the bread and drizzle mole sauce over the top.

FIXES FOR ONE

Sometimes you just need a bite of something delicious to get you through to 5 pm. We've compiled a bunch of recipes that the IQS Team regularly whips up when we get desperate.

PEANUT BUTTER PROTEIN CRUNCHIES

Peanut butter addicts rejoice, this recipe is for YOU. A little crunch,
a lot of peanut butter and a coating of chocolate. Heaven!

MAKES 14

PREPARATION TIME
30 minutes

COOKING TIME
2 minutes

½ cup (85 g) 'activated groaties'
(activated buckwheat groats)

½ cup (50 g) protein powder or
almond meal

1 tablespoon coconut cream

½ cup (90 g) peanut butter

60 g dark chocolate (85% cocoa),
chopped into small pieces

1. In a bowl combine activated groaties, protein powder, coconut cream
   and peanut butter.

2. Roll into small balls. Sit in the freezer on a tray lined with baking paper
   to set for about 30 minutes.

3. Melt chocolate over a double boiler, ensuring the chocolate doesn't seize.

4. Remove balls from the freezer and coat in melted chocolate. Place back
   in the fridge to set. Serve.

> **TRICKY TIP**
>
> These protein balls are best served straight from the fridge.

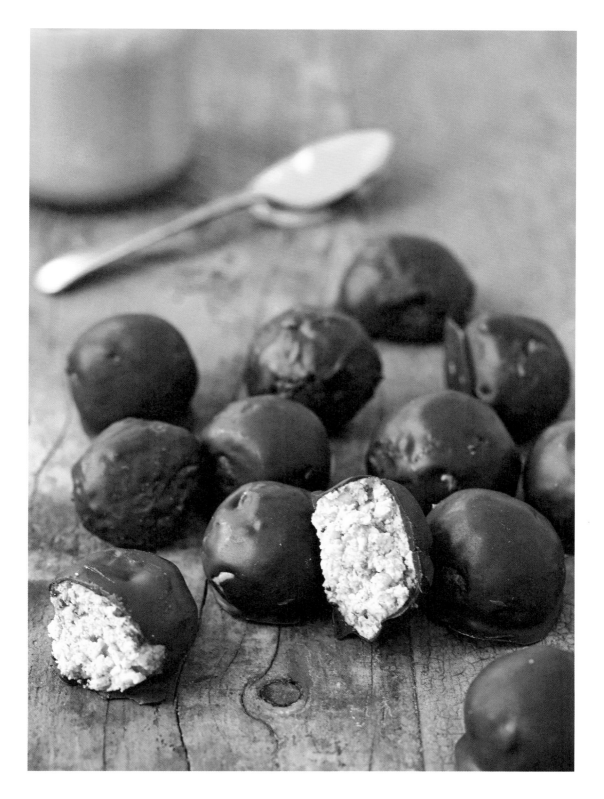

ESPRESSO TRUFFLES

These truffles are a great dinner party treat. Serve up a few on a plate and let your guests devour them one by one.

MAKES 14

PREPARATION TIME
2 hours

COOKING TIME
5 minutes

1 cup (250 ml) Basic Raw Chocolate (see page 13)

1 tablespoon instant coffee granules

½ tablespoon boiling water

¼ cup (60 ml) coconut cream

2 teaspoons granulated stevia or 1 tablespoon rice malt syrup

raw cacao powder to decorate, optional

1. Lay out 16 mini paper cases or a silicon ice cube tray.

2. Combine all of the ingredients in a small saucepan over a low heat. Be sure to stir well so the rice malt syrup is evenly distributed.

3. Remove from heat and pour mixture into silicon moulds or paper cases.

4. Place truffles in the fridge or freezer for up to 2 hours until set.

5. To serve, pop out truffles from mould and sift raw cacao over the top, if you like.

> **TRICKY TIP**
>
> To jazz these up use moulds in various shapes. Serve a few after dinner.

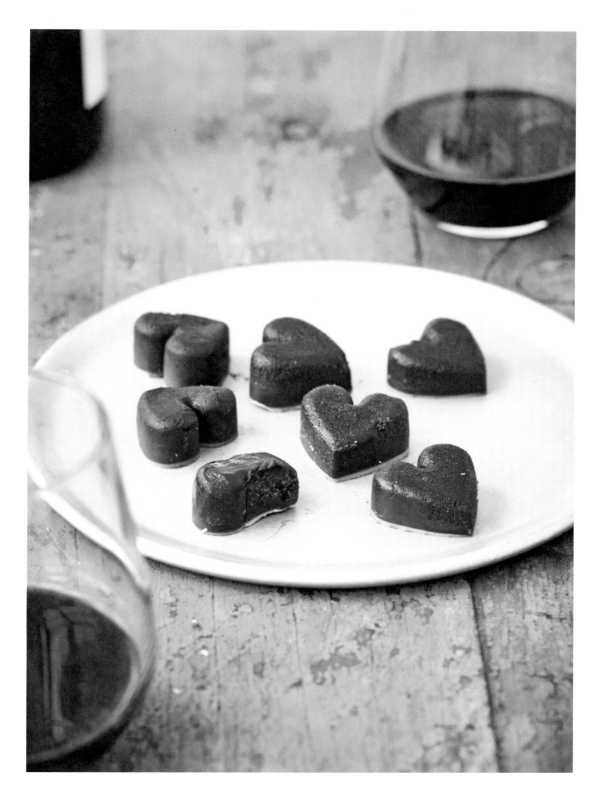

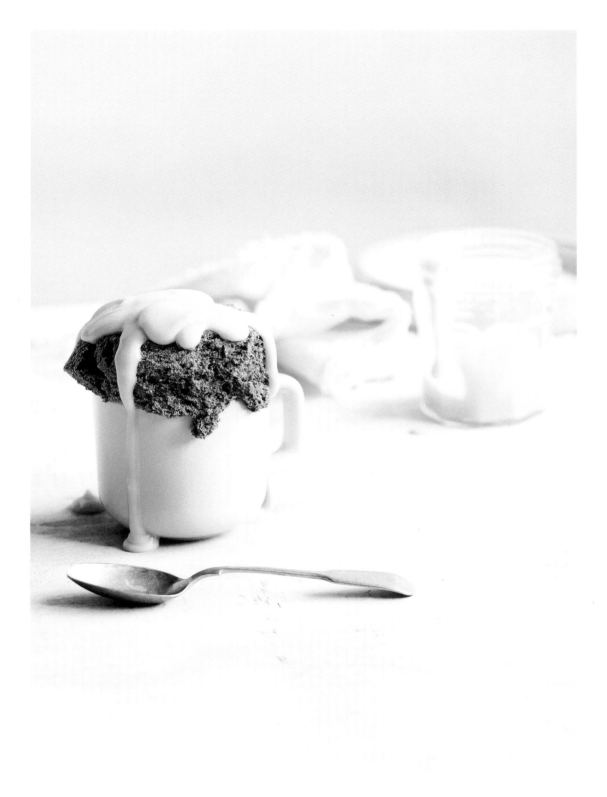

CHOCOLATE AND CINNAMON BUN MUGGIN WITH CARAMEL AND COCONUT ICING

This delicious muggin came about at 3pm one afternoon in the IQS office. We were all craving something a little special to get us through to dinner. Five minutes later, we were devouring this sweet 'n' spiced treat. The satisfied chorus from the office meant we had to include it in the cookbook!

SERVES 1

PREPARATION TIME
3 minutes

COOKING TIME
2 minutes

3 tablespoons coconut flour

2 teaspoons raw cacao powder

½ teaspoon baking powder

1 teaspoon ground cinnamon

½ teaspoon allspice

½ teaspoon vanilla powder or extract, optional

2 tablespoons coconut milk (or milk of your choice)

1 egg

ICING

½ tablespoon Gooey Caramel Sauce (see page 162)

½ tablespoon Coconut Butter (see page 156)

1 tablespoon coconut milk

1. Make the icing by combining all of the ingredients in a small bowl or mug.

2. Combine remaining ingredients in a mug and stir until mixed completely. Microwave for 2 minutes. Pour icing over the top and serve.

> TRICKY TIP
>
> To make this vegan, omit the caramel sauce.

COCONUT BALLS

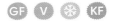

MAKES 14

PREPARATION TIME
1 hour 30 minutes

COOKING TIME
5 minutes

FILLING

2½ cups (190 g) unsweetened shredded coconut

2 tablespoons rice malt syrup

2 tablespoons coconut oil, melted

¼ cup (60 ml) coconut milk

CHOCOLATE COATING

1 cup (250 ml) Basic Raw Chocolate (see page 13) or 1 cup (225 g) store-bought dark (85% cocoa) chocolate

1. Line a baking tray with baking paper. Add all the filling ingredients to the food processor. Pulse until mixture comes together but still has texture. Roll tablespoons of the mixture into round balls and freeze for at least an hour.

2. Meanwhile make Basic Raw Chocolate or melt store-bought chocolate over a double boiler, being careful not to seize the chocolate. Remove the coconut balls from the freezer and roll them in the melted chocolate so they are completely coated.

3. Place balls on a tray and sit in the fridge to set before serving.

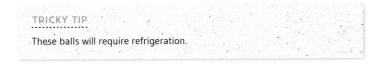

TRICKY TIP

These balls will require refrigeration.

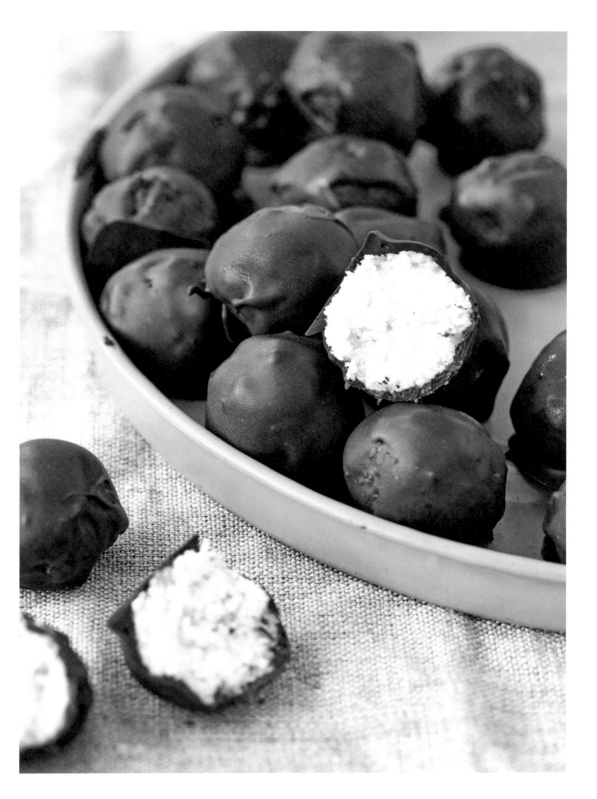

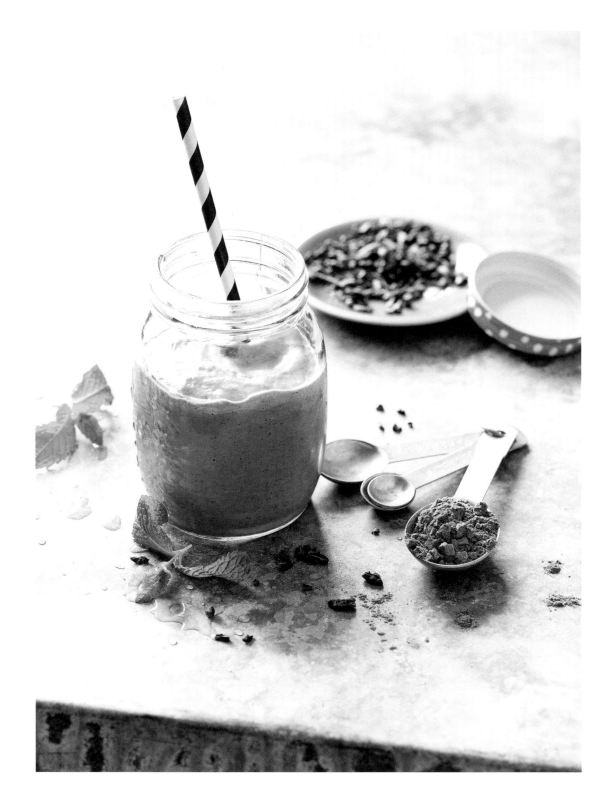

CHOCOLATE CHIP
+ MINT WHIP

Cacao nibs make the perfect choc chips. They're completely dairy- and sugar-free and taste great paired with some fresh mint leaves, like in this green smoothie.

SERVES 2

PREPARATION TIME
5 minutes

1½ cups (375 ml) almond milk

1 small avocado

1 cup (50 g) mint leaves

¼ cup (25 g) protein powder
of your choice

2 tablespoons green powder,
optional

pinch of stevia granules,
to taste

½ cup (120 ml) ice cubes

2 tablespoons cacao nibs

1. Throw all the ingredients, except the cacao nibs, into a blender and blend until smooth. Toss in the nibs and blend for an extra few pulses. Pour into two glasses and serve cold.

FUDGY PROTEIN BITES

The protein powder in these chocolatey bites gives a wonderfully chewy texture and the way the ingredients naturally settle means the chia and rice malt syrup form a caramel-like base on the bottom, followed by a fudgy centre covered in chocolate. Seriously good stuff.

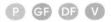

SERVES 25

PREPARATION TIME
1 hour 5 minutes

1½ cups (375 ml) Basic Raw Chocolate (see page 13), melted

½ cup (80 g) chia seeds

⅓ cup (40 g) maca powder, optional (if not using maca, add a little extra protein powder)

¾ cup (75 g) vanilla protein powder

1. Combine all ingredients and pour immediately into silicon moulds or cupcake cases (mini or standard). Place in the fridge or freezer for at least 1 hour to harden.

> **TRICKY TIP**
>
> Add ¼ teaspoon vanilla powder if you're using a natural protein powder.

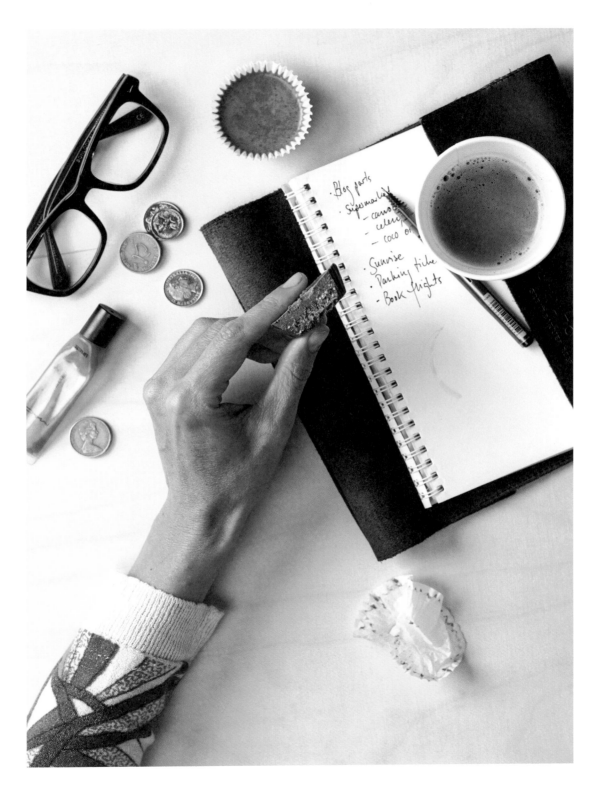

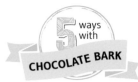

5 ways with CHOCOLATE BARK

THE BEAUTY OF CHOCOLATE BARK is you can make up any combination you like using the ingredients you have. We've listed five of our favourites below.

1 CINNAMON AND ALMOND CRUNCH

SERVES 6–8

PREPARATION TIME
1 hour 5 minutes

1 cup (250 ml) Basic Raw Chocolate (see page 13), melted

1 teaspoon ground cinnamon

½ cup (70 g) almonds, roughly chopped

1. Line a tray or plate (with a lip, so the mixture doesn't spill) with baking paper. Combine Basic Raw Chocolate, cinnamon and half of the almonds.

2. Pour mixture onto tray and scatter with remaining almonds. Sit in the fridge for at least 1 hour before serving.

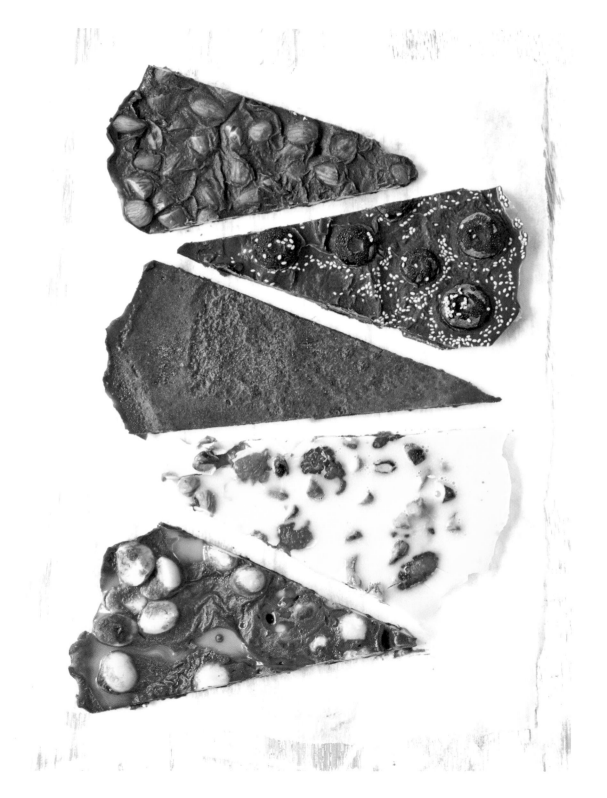

2 SUPERFOOD BARK

SERVES 6–8

PREPARATION TIME
1 hour 5 minutes

1 cup (250 ml) Basic Raw Chocolate (see page 13), melted

2 teaspoons maca powder

1 tablespoon chia seeds

½ cup (50 g) blueberries

1. Line a tray or plate (with a lip, so the mixture doesn't spill) with baking paper. Combine Basic Raw Chocolate, maca, chia seeds and half of the blueberries.

2. Pour mixture onto tray and scatter with remaining blueberries. Sit in the fridge for at least 1 hour before serving.

3 CHILLI CHOC

SERVES 6–8

PREPARATION TIME
1 hour 5 minutes

1 cup (250 ml) Basic Raw Chocolate (see page 13), melted

½ teaspoon of dried chilli powder + extra for dusting

1. Line a tray or plate (with a lip, so the mixture doesn't spill) with baking paper. Combine Basic Raw Chocolate and chilli powder.

2. Pour mixture onto tray and scatter with extra chilli powder. Sit in the fridge for at least 1 hour before serving.

4 WHITE CHRISTMAS BARK

SERVES 6–8

PREPARATION TIME
1 hour 5 minutes

½ cup (115 g) raw cacao butter,
buttons or shavings

½ cup (100 g) coconut oil

¼ cup (60 ml) rice malt syrup

½ cup (60 g) raspberries,
roughly chopped

¼ cup (40 g) pistachios,
roughly chopped

1. Line a tray or plate (with a lip, so the mixture doesn't spill) with baking paper. Combine cacao butter, coconut oil and rice malt syrup in a small saucepan over a medium heat.

2. Pour mixture onto tray and scatter with raspberries and pistachios. Sit in the fridge for at least 1 hour before serving.

5 MACADAMIA 'N' CARAMEL SWIRL

SERVES 6–8

PREPARATION TIME
1 hour 5 minutes

1 cup (250 ml) Basic Raw Chocolate
(see page 13), melted

½ cup (60 g) macadamias,
roughly chopped

¼ cup (60 ml) Gooey Caramel
Sauce (see page 162)

1. Line a tray or plate (with a lip, so the mixture doesn't spill) with baking paper. In a bowl combine Basic Raw Chocolate and half of the macadamias.

2. Pour mixture onto tray and scatter with remaining macadamias and drizzle Gooey Caramel Sauce over the top. Sit in the fridge for at least 1 hour before serving.

SWEET POTATO, DARK CHOCOLATE + SEA SALT CHIPS

SERVES 4

PREPARATION TIME
5 minutes

COOKING TIME
10 minutes

coconut oil, for frying

1 large sweet potato, thinly sliced (the thinner the chip, the better the final outcome – a mandolin works well for this)

60 g dark chocolate (85–90% cocoa), chopped into even-sized pieces

sea salt, to taste

1. Line a baking tray or plate with kitchen paper.

2. Add enough coconut oil into a medium frying pan until it is 1 cm deep. Heat until bubbling. Using a slotted spoon, carefully lower chips into coconut oil to shallow fry. Do not overcrowd the pan. Turn once and remove from pan to drain on kitchen paper. Repeat process until all of the chips have been fried.

3. Line a baking tray or plate with baking paper. Melt chocolate over a double boiler or in a microwave (for about 30 seconds) until smooth.

4. Dip fried sweet potato into chocolate and place on baking paper. Sprinkle with sea salt. Set in the fridge until chocolate hardens before serving.

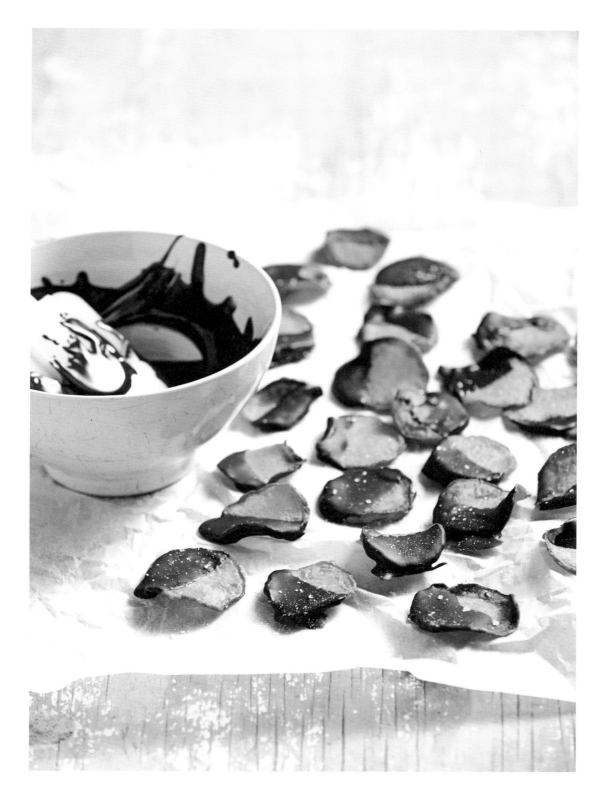

TOP DECK FUDGE

This chewy fudge is a favourite at IQS HQ because it's a breeze to whip up and only has a handful of ingredients. Next time you need a chocolate hit look no further.

MAKES 40

PREPARATION TIME
40 minutes

COOKING TIME
5 minutes

¼ cup (50 g) coconut oil

½ cup (115 g) cashew butter

¼ cup (25 g) raw cacao powder

¼ cup (25 g) chocolate protein powder

1 tablespoon rice malt syrup

pinch of sea salt

¼ cup (60 ml) coconut cream + ½ cup (120 ml) coconut cream chilled in the refrigerator

1. Line a small plastic container (a small lunchbox works well) or loaf tin with baking paper. In a saucepan on a low heat combine all the ingredients but the chilled coconut cream. Stir until smooth.

2. Pour mixture into lined container and sit in the freezer for at least 30 minutes or until firm to the touch. Remove from the freezer and spoon chilled coconut cream over the top. Smooth with the back of a spoon.

3. Place fudge back in the freezer until coconut cream sets. Slice into squares and serve.

> **TRICKY TIP**
>
> You can control the portion sizes by pouring the mixture into an ice cube tray. Simply pop out one cube when you fancy a treat.

SAME-SAME
BUT DIFFERENT

From Ferrero Rochers to caramel slice,
we've IQS-ified all your favourites!

SALTED CARAMEL SLICE

This is one of the most popular recipes IQS has ever created. We promise, you'll never need a bite of regular caramel slice ever again.

SERVES 36

PREPARATION TIME
6 hours

COOKING TIME
25 minutes

BASE

1 cup (115 g) gluten-free flour

½ cup (50 g) almond meal

110 g butter (diced into small cubes)

4 tablespoons rice malt syrup

GOOEY CARAMEL SAUCE

½ cup (120 ml) rice malt syrup

100 g butter (diced into small cubes)

pinch of sea salt

½ cup (120 ml) full-fat coconut cream

CHOCOLATE GANACHE TOPPING

¾ cup (175 ml) full-fat coconut cream

80 g dark chocolate (85% cocoa, but you can use 90% if you prefer)

BASE

1. Preheat oven to 180°C (gas 4). Line a 22 cm square brownie tin with baking paper.

2. Mix all of the base ingredients together until combined. Press mixture firmly into the prepared tin so base is even. Bake for 15–20 minutes, or until golden. Remove from oven and set aside to cool completely.

GOOEY CARAMEL SAUCE

1. Heat rice malt syrup in a pan until bubbling vigorously. If you have a sugar thermometer it should reach 135°C. If you don't have a thermometer, cook the syrup for 13 minutes until syrup has reduced down. The mixture should be thick, drippy and coat the back of a spoon lightly.

2. Add butter and salt and stir over medium heat until combined. Remove from heat and slowly add coconut cream, stirring until combined. Pour caramel into a bowl and sit in the freezer until thick for 2 hours.

3. Once thick, pour caramel on top of the biscuit base and spread over the base with the back of a spoon. Refrigerate for a further 2 hours or until set. The longer you leave it in the fridge the better the final product will be.

CHOCOLATE GANACHE TOPPING

1. Heat the coconut cream in a saucepan until it simmers. Turn off the heat and pour into a separate bowl, add chocolate pieces and stir gently until melted and silky. Allow to cool for 5–10 minutes until mixture thickens but still pours.

2. Remove the set base from the refrigerator and pour ganache over the top. Smooth with the back of a spoon or a pastry knife. Return to the refrigerator and set for at least 2 hours before serving. Store in the fridge or freezer until ready to serve.

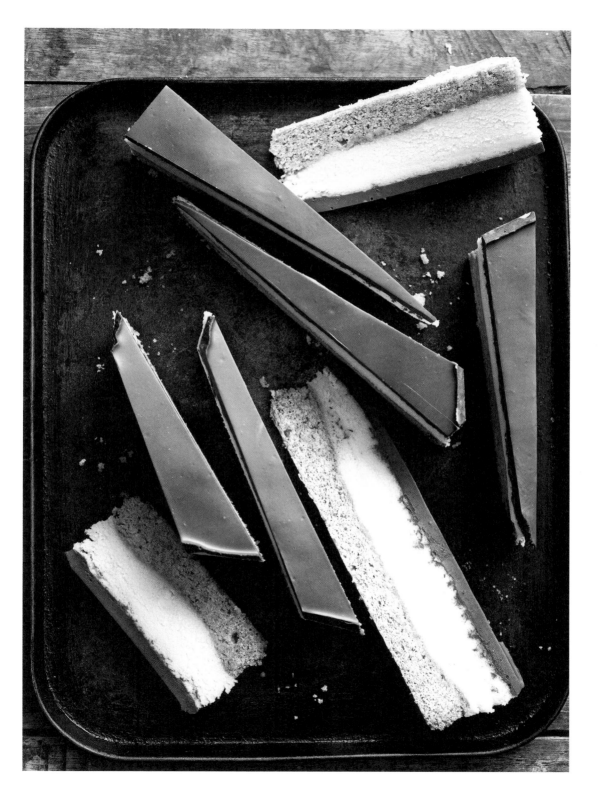

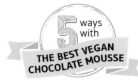

VEGAN CHOCOLATE MOUSSE

Running low on time? This Vegan Chocolate Mousse can be whipped up as a special dessert in minutes and left in the fridge for hours without any extra effort needed. Pick a flavour variation to make it extra special.

SERVES 4–6

PREPARATION TIME
3 hours

1 x 400 ml can coconut cream

½ cup (50 g) raw cacao powder

¼ cup (60 ml) rice malt syrup

¼ cup (40 g) chia seeds

cacao nibs, optional

1. Place all the ingredients except the cacao nibs in a large mixing bowl and whisk together until well combined and smooth. Pour into 4–6 serving glasses. Sprinkle with cacao nibs if desired.

2. Chill in the fridge for at least 3 hours, or until firm.

VARIATIONS

Jaffa Joy

Add 1 tablespoon orange zest, and the juice of ½ an orange to the mixture in Step 1.

Choco Mint

Add 1 teaspoon peppermint essence or ⅓ cup (15 g) very finely chopped mint leaves to the mixture in Step 1.

Salted Caramel

Gently stir through ¼ cup (60 ml) Gooey Caramel Sauce (see page 162) before setting in the fridge. Sprinkle sea salt on top.

Raspberry Rush

Add ½ cup (60 g) frozen, thawed and mashed raspberries in Step 1. Top with extra raspberries.

Turkish Rose

Add 1 teaspoon rosewater in Step 1. Top mousse with pistachios and rose petals, then serve.

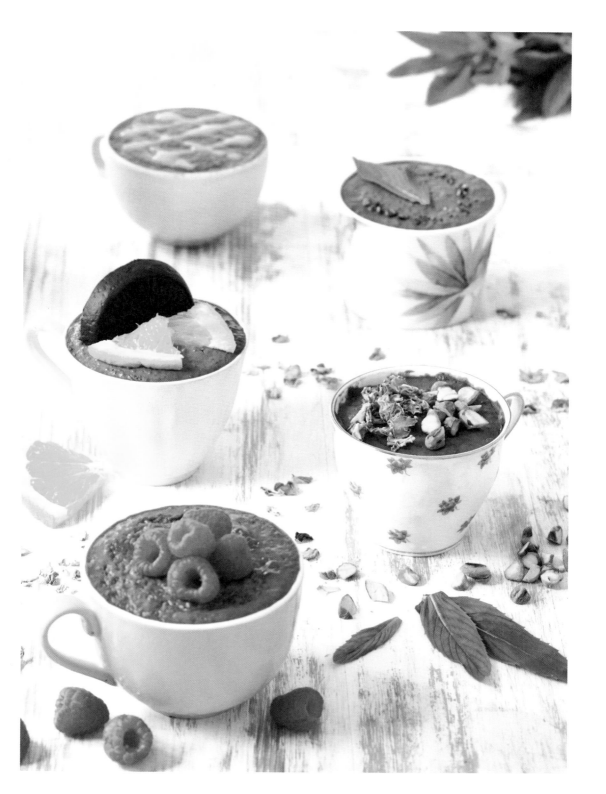

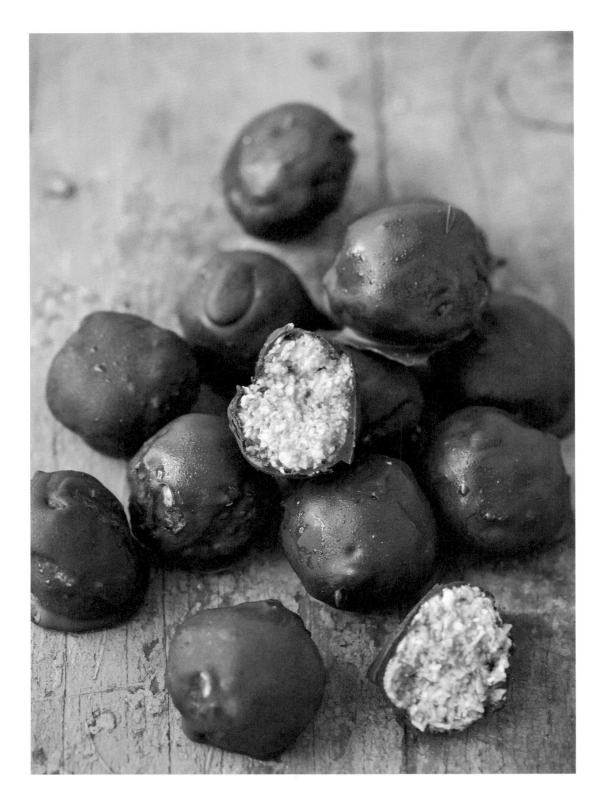

NOT QUITE
CHERRY RIPE BITES

*These little morsels have everything you need in one bite:
low-fructose fruit, good fat and chocolate. Tick, tick, tick!*

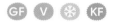

MAKES 12

PREPARATION TIME
1 hour 30 minutes

COOKING TIME
5 minutes

FILLING

1¼ cups (115 g) unsweetened shredded coconut

1 tablespoon rice malt syrup

1 tablespoon coconut oil, melted

1½ tablespoons coconut milk

1 teaspoon vanilla powder or extract, optional

½ cup (60 g) raspberries (fresh or frozen)

CHOCOLATE COATING

1 cup (250 ml) Basic Raw Chocolate (see page 13) or 1 cup (225 g) store-bought dark chocolate (85% cocoa)

1. Line a baking tray with baking paper. Add all the filling ingredients to the food processor. Pulse until mixture comes together but still has texture. Roll tablespoons of the mixture into round balls, place on a baking tray and freeze for at least 1 hour.

2. Meanwhile make Basic Raw Chocolate or melt store-bought chocolate over a double boiler being careful not to seize the chocolate. Remove the coconut balls from the freezer and roll them in the melted chocolate so they are completely coated.

3. Place balls on a tray and sit in the fridge to set before serving.

> **TRICKY TIP**
> These balls will require refrigeration.

HAZELNUT CHOCOLATE BOMBS

There is something about these chocolates that reminds us of celebration. Perhaps it's the gold foil, or the fact that the ads saturate our TV screens at special times of the year. Now you can enjoy them without sugar – hurrah!

A caveat: If it's hot, these can be tricky to perfect. They require patience, a cool kitchen (temperature wise, stylish is optional) and a good fridge. The end result is definitely worth the effort, but if you want a quick and easy version, we suggest you make the Hazelnut Chocolate Slice (see opposite page).

MAKES 20

PREPARATION TIME
3 hours

COOKING TIME
15 minutes

SHELL

4 cups (500 g) hazelnuts

200 g dark chocolate
(85% cocoa)

FILLING

1 cup (125 g) hazelnuts

¼ cup (50 g) coconut oil

¼ cup (60 ml) rice malt syrup

1–2 tablespoons coconut milk

¼ cup (25 g) raw cacao powder

1 teaspoon vanilla powder
or extract, optional

HAZELNUT CHOCOLATE BOMBS (ADVANCED OPTION)

1. Preheat oven to 180°C (gas 4). Place all hazelnuts (including ones for the filling) on an oven tray. Cook for 8–10 minutes until roasted and skins are beginning to fall off. Cool slightly. Rub skins off using a tea towel.

2. Place one cup (125 g) of hazelnuts and remaining filling ingredients in a food processor. Process until smooth.

3. Refrigerate for 30 minutes. Meanwhile place half of the remaining hazelnuts in a food processor and process until finely chopped. Place on a plate.

4. Roll filling mixture into balls and insert a whole hazelnut inside each ball working quickly so they don't melt. Place back in refrigerator for 1 hour.

5. Simmer some water in a saucepan on the stove top. Place a heatproof bowl on top and gently melt the chocolate (or melt chocolate in the microwave).

6. Dip refrigerated balls into melted chocolate to coat, then sprinkle with chopped hazelnuts and place back in refrigerator on a tray lined with baking paper. Allow to set for at least 2 hours.

SEE OPPOSITE PAGE FOR AN EASIER OPTION >

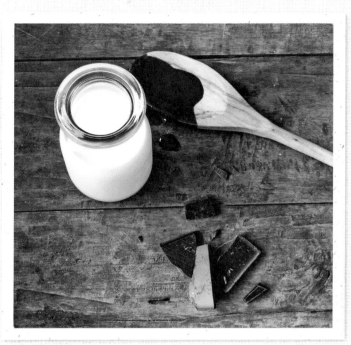

HAZELNUT CHOCOLATE SLICE (EASIER OPTION)

1. Follow Steps 1 and 2 in the advanced option.

2. Line a shallow baking tray or a loaf tin with baking paper extending paper over sides of the tin.

3. Press filling mixture into base of tray. Insert half remaining hazelnuts intermittently throughout filling. Refrigerate for at least 1 hour.

4. Meanwhile chop remaining hazelnuts in a food processor and melt chocolate as per instructions in Step 5 of the advanced option.

5. Pour melted chocolate evenly over filling in tray. Sprinkle with chopped hazelnuts and refrigerate for at least 1 hour or until set.

6. Cut into squares and serve.

CHEWY PEANUT
CARAMEL BARS

This is Sarah's favourite recipe from the whole cookbook. It's got the perfect combination of sweetness and saltiness. Making these can be a process but it's well worth it, just for the 'oooh's' and 'ahhh's' when presented to friends and family.

SERVES 20

PREPARATION TIME
4 hours

COOKING TIME
10 minutes

'NOUGAT' BASE

½ cup (120 ml) coconut cream

2 tablespoons rice malt syrup

pinch of sea salt

1 teaspoon vanilla powder
or extract, optional

5 tablespoons coconut flour
+ extra if needed

½ cup (115 g) peanut or cashew butter

FILLING

½ cup (120 ml) Gooey Caramel Sauce
(see page 162)

¼ cup (40 g) peanuts, roughly chopped

CHOCOLATE COATING

100 g dark chocolate (85% cocoa)
or 1½ cups (375 ml) Basic Raw
Chocolate (see page 13)

1. Line a loaf tin with baking paper. Combine all ingredients for the base in a bowl until mixture comes together and forms a very soft dough. You may need to add more coconut flour to achieve the right consistency.

2. Spoon mixture into lined tin and freeze for 1–2 hours or until firm to the touch. Remove from the freezer and cover with Gooey Caramel Sauce. Sprinkle with chopped peanuts and slice base into 20 even pieces. Place back in the freezer for a further hour to set again.

3. In the meantime line a baking tray with baking paper. Melt the store-bought chocolate or make the Basic Raw Chocolate over a double boiler. Remove the bars from the freezer and dip each bar in the chocolate. Place onto the lined tray and put back in the freezer until ready to serve.

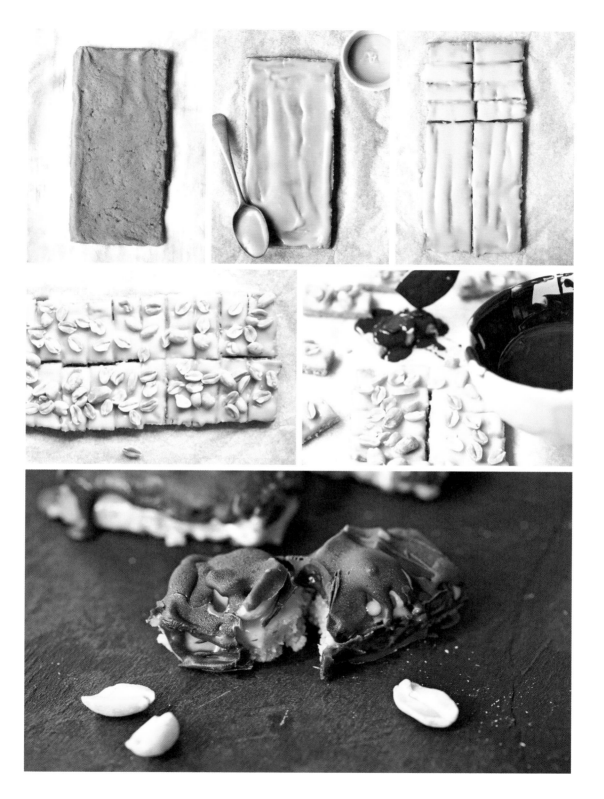

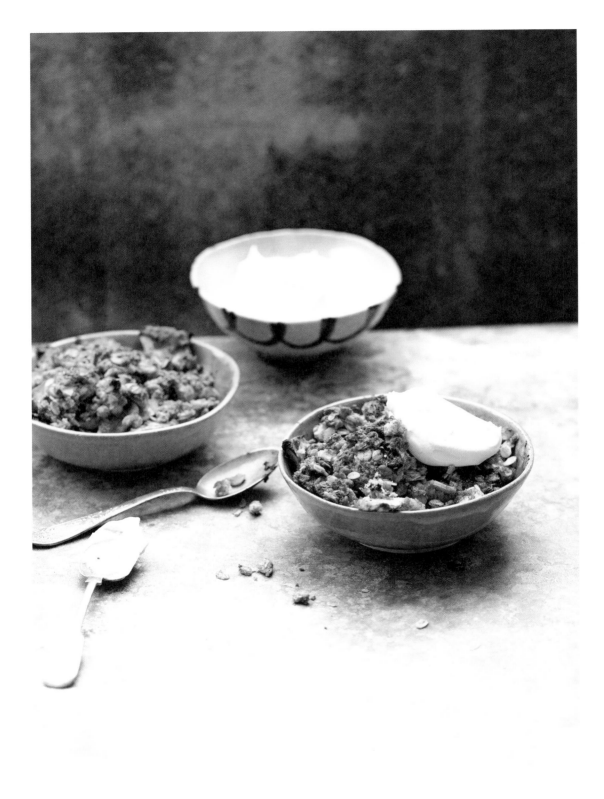

APPLE 'N'
CHOC-CHIP CRUMBLE

Nothing beats wholesome apple pie with a crunchy baked crumble.
Except for maybe chocolate.

SERVES 2

PREPARATION TIME
10 minutes

COOKING TIME
35 minutes

APPLE FILLING

1 apple, peeled and roughly chopped

2 teaspoons lemon juice

1 teaspoon rice malt syrup

1 teaspoon coconut flour

1 teaspoon ground cinnamon

½ teaspoon ground nutmeg

CRUMBLE TOPPING

1 tablespoon butter, softened

1 tablespoon rice malt syrup

½ teaspoon vanilla powder or extract, optional

¼ cup (25 g) almond meal

¼ teaspoon ground cinnamon

pinch of sea salt

¼ cup (25 g) gluten-free oats

2 squares dark chocolate (85% cocoa), finely chopped

natural full-fat yoghurt or cream, to serve

1. Preheat the oven to 180°C (gas 4). Have two 9 cm-wide ramekins ready.

2. To make the filling, in a large bowl mix all the ingredients together. Divide between the two ramekins and bake for 15 minutes. Let cool while you make the topping.

3. To make the topping, combine all the ingredients except the yoghurt or cream in a bowl. The mixture will be crumbly.

4. Top the cooked apples with the crumble mixture. Bake for 15 minutes or until the top is golden brown. Cool for 15 minutes before serving warm. Top with yoghurt or cream.

MISS MARZIPAN'S JAVA CHIP FRAPPU-CHIA-NO

Recipe by Marisa of missmarzipan.com
This certainly trumps those syrupy, sweet monstrosities you get from coffee chains.
Try it out and see if you notice a difference.

SERVES 2

PREPARATION TIME
25 minutes

SMOOTHIE BASE

1 cup (250 ml) almond milk (or milk of your choice)

2½ tablespoons chia seeds

2 tablespoons almond meal

200 ml cold coffee

½ teaspoon vanilla powder or extract, optional

½ tablespoon rice malt syrup

CHOCOLATE SAUCE

2 tablespoons coconut oil

2 tablespoons raw cacao powder

2 tablespoons rice malt syrup

TO SERVE

300 ml crushed ice (or more if you like)

1 cup (250 ml) Whipped Coconut Cream (see page 158)

raw cacao nibs

1. Pour the almond milk into a blender. Stir the chia seeds into the almond milk and allow them to soak for 20 minutes.

2. Meanwhile, make the chocolate sauce by combining the sauce ingredients in a small pan and heating through while stirring over a low heat. Remove from heat and let cool (it will thicken up a little after cooling).

3. Add the remaining smoothie base ingredients to the blender plus 2 tablespoons of the chocolate sauce (reserving the rest for serving). Blitz the mix until well combined and smooth.

4. Divide smoothie between two large glasses and pop in the fridge (they can be left overnight, if you want to make them in advance).

5. When ready to serve, add enough crushed ice to fill each smoothie glass, gently stirring through to combine.

6. Top each smoothie with whipped coconut cream, cacao nibs and a drizzle of the remaining sauce.

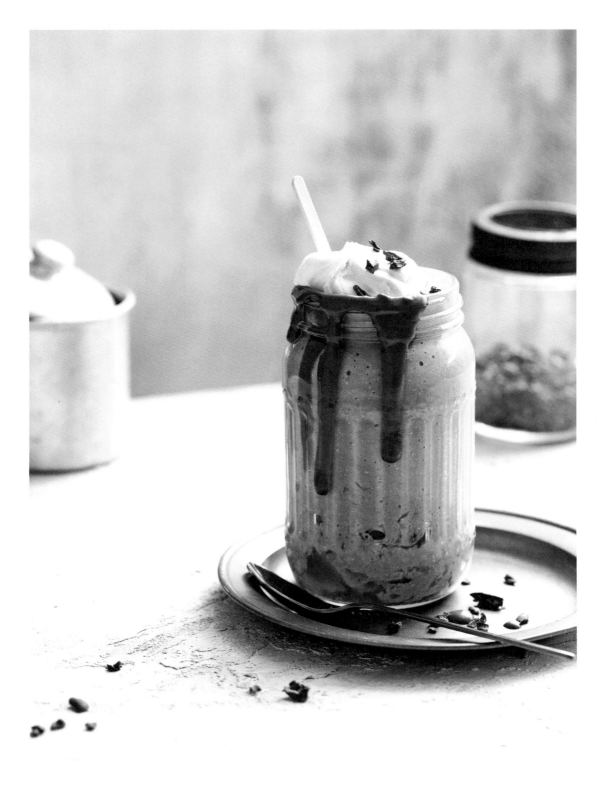

CAMPFIRE S'MORES

This is the best sandwich you'll ever eat, you can be sure. Everyone will be wanting s'more of these.

MAKES 4–6

PREPARATION TIME
15 minutes

COOKING TIME
45 minutes

'GRAHAM' CRACKERS

¼ cup (25 g) almond meal

½ cup (60 g) coconut flour

pinch of sea salt

¼ teaspoon baking powder

1 teaspoon ground cinnamon

½ teaspoon vanilla powder or extract, optional

¼ cup (50 g) coconut oil, melted

2 tablespoons rice malt syrup

1 egg

CHOCOLATE

1 square of dark chocolate (85% cocoa), per s'more

'MARSHMALLOW' CENTRES

2 large egg whites, about 4 tablespoons

2 tablespoons rice malt syrup

pinch of sea salt

1 teaspoon rosewater

1 teaspoon iced water

1. Preheat oven to 180°C (gas 4). Line a baking tray with baking paper.

2. To make the crackers, combine all dry ingredients in a small bowl. Place the wet ingredients in a large bowl and whisk to combine. Add dry ingredients and mix until well combined. Roll mixture out on a floured surface into a rectangle (about 5-mm thick). Cut into squares (about 3 cm square) but no need to pull them apart. Place mixture on a tray and bake in the oven for 10–12 minutes. Set aside to cool. Reduce oven to the lowest temperature setting, about 110°C (gas ¼).

3. To make the 'Marshmallow' Centres, bring 5 cm of water to a simmer in a saucepan. In a heatproof mixing bowl, combine the egg whites, rice malt syrup and pinch of salt. Place the bowl over the simmering water, being careful not to let it touch the water. Whisk the egg whites constantly for 3–5 minutes, until they are warm to the touch.

4. Remove from the heat, then transfer the mixing bowl to a stand mixer or use a hand-held beater. Add in the rosewater and immediately begin whipping on high. Pour in the teaspoon of iced water, then keep beating on high until thick and glossy, about 5 minutes.

5. Line a baking tray with baking paper and place small dollops of meringue on the tray. Bake for about 20–30 minutes or until semi solid to touch. You want them half cooked so they are a little chewy.

6. To serve: make a sandwich with the biscuits, marshmallow and chocolate, then wrap in foil and bake at 180°C (gas 4) for 5–10 minutes or until chocolate has melted. This can also be done around the edge of a campfire.

CHOCOLATE 'N' SPICE PUMPKIN PIE

*Don't be impatient when making this pie. It's much better when it's cooked properly
(it should look like a baked custard when you remove it from the oven). Also, be sure
to leave it to cool for a good few hours (to allow it to set right). In fact, it's actually nicer
the next day when it has set fully. It also works well frozen and thawed just a little.*

SERVES 12

PREPARATION TIME
1 hour 30 minutes

COOKING TIME
1 hour

CRUST

60 g butter, melted

2 cups (200 g) almond or hazelnut
meal, or a combination of both, or
LSA (linseed, sunflower seed
and almond blend)

1 teaspoon sea salt

FILLING

3 eggs

¼ cup (60 ml) rice malt syrup

1½ cups (375 ml) Pumpkin Purée
(see page 166)

¼ cup (25 g) raw cacao powder

¾ cup (175 ml) cream + extra
to serve

1 tablespoon grated
fresh ginger

1 teaspoon ground cinnamon

¼ teaspoon ground nutmeg

¼ teaspoon ground cloves

1 teaspoon sea salt

1–2 tablespoons arrowroot
or tapioca flour

natural full-fat yoghurt or
cream, to serve

1. Preheat the oven to 180°C (gas 4). To make the crust, combine the
    melted butter, nut meal and salt in a bowl. Mix well. The more you work
    the mixture the better it will turn out.

2. Press the mixture into the bottom and sides of a 22 cm pie dish to
    make a pie crust. If there isn't quite enough mixture, throw in a bit
    more of both butter and meal. Bake in the oven for 5–8 minutes until
    it just starts to turn golden. Remove from the oven and allow base to
    cool fully, at least an hour.

3. To make the filling, cream the eggs and syrup, then blend in the rest of
    the ingredients until the mixture is the consistency of thin custard. If it's
    a bit too runny, add extra arrowroot.

4. Gently pour the filling into the cold crust and bake for 45–55 minutes
    or until the centre of the pie is 'set' (when it starts to crack away from
    the base a little). Remove from the oven and cool completely before
    putting in the fridge. Serve with yoghurt or cream.

MEXICAN HOT CHOCOLATE

SERVES 2

PREPARATION TIME
2 minutes

COOKING TIME
10 minutes

2 cups (500 ml) coconut milk

1 teaspoon ground cinnamon
or 1 cinnamon stick

½ teaspoon vanilla powder
or extract, optional

¼ teaspoon ground nutmeg

pinch of cayenne pepper

pinch of chilli powder

1½ tablespoons raw
cacao powder

1 teaspoon rice malt syrup

2 squares dark chocolate
(85% cocoa)

1. Combine all the ingredients except for the dark chocolate in a small
   pan over a medium heat.

2. Bring milk to the boil then reduce to a low simmer. Cover and cook
   for 10 minutes. Remove cinnamon stick (or leave in for decoration).
   Serve with a square of dark chocolate plonked into each mug.

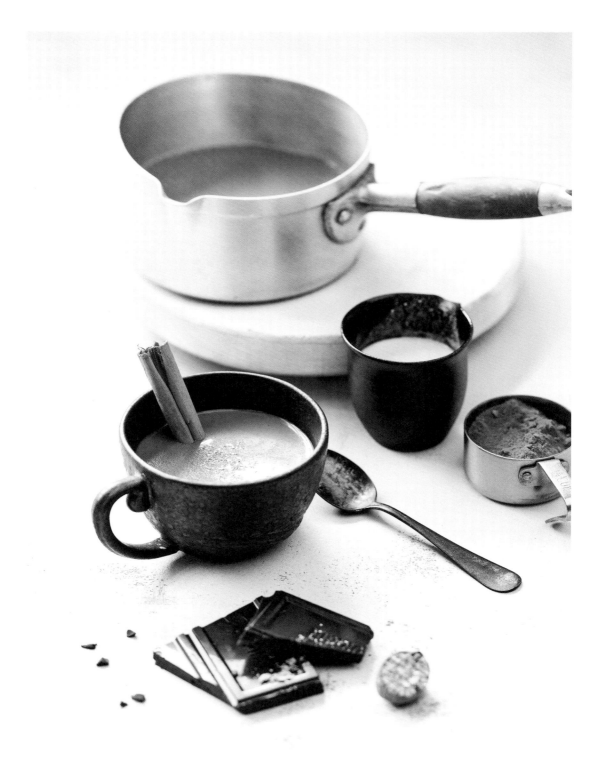

AVOCADO CHOCOLATE MOUSSE

Love chocolate mousse but don't eat it anymore since quitting the white stuff?
We have the perfect solution – avocado! Avo makes these desserts silky smooth
and when mixed with chia seeds, helps them firm up.

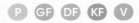

SERVES 4

PREPARATION TIME
2 hours 5 minutes

2 avocados

125 ml coconut cream, chilled
(it needs to be firm)

⅓ cup (30 g) raw cacao powder

1 tablespoon chia seeds

1 teaspoon granulated stevia

¼ teaspoon vanilla powder

½ teaspoon ground cinnamon

pinch of sea salt

1. Place all ingredients in a blender and blitz until smooth. Scoop the mousse into small serving dishes, such as antique teacups, and put in the fridge to chill for at least 2 hours. Serve.

CHOCOLATE NUT BUTTER CUPS

You know those junky peanut butter cups you can buy? Well, these are same-same-but-way-better. We've provided a number of variations for the filling, too.

SERVES 10

PREPARATION TIME
50 minutes

½ cup (100 g) coconut oil, melted

½ cup (50 g) raw cacao powder

1 tablespoon rice malt syrup

2 tablespoons coconut cream

¼ cup (50 g) peanut butter, smooth

pinch of sea salt

1. Arrange small paper cases on a tray. Whisk together the coconut oil and cacao powder until smooth, then stir in the rice malt syrup and coconut cream. Pour a thin layer into the bottom of the paper cases. Place in the freezer for 5 minutes.

2. Remove chocolates from the freezer and spoon ⅓ teaspoon peanut butter into each one. Pour the remaining chocolate mixture on top and scatter sea salt over. Place in the fridge to set for 30 minutes (or, if you're short of time, freeze them).

3. Once set, eat straight from the fridge – these will melt at room temperature.

VARIATIONS

Coconut Butter Cups

Make a coconut version by using a small ball of Coconut Butter (see page 156) instead of the nut spread.

Peppermint Patties

Add a few drops of peppermint oil (to taste) to small balls of coconut butter instead of the nut spread.

Pumpkin Protein Cups

Mix together 4 tablespoons each of Pumpkin Purée (see page 166), almond butter and vanilla protein powder, with 2 teaspoons coconut oil and ½ teaspoon each cinnamon and allspice. Put mixture in the freezer for a couple of hours. Once mixture is hard enough to handle, roll into ⅓ teaspoon balls and use instead of the nut spread.

CHOCOLATE-TIPPED MACAROONS

Filled with good fats and protein, these coco-nutty macaroons not only taste super delicious, but are great for your afternoon energy slump.

SERVES 12

PREPARATION TIME
2 hours 15 minutes

COOKING TIME
15 minutes

3 large egg whites

⅓ cup (75 ml) rice malt syrup

1½ cups (125 g) shredded coconut

1 cup (175 g) cooked quinoa

pinch of sea salt

50 g dark chocolate (85–90% cocoa)

1 tablespoon coconut oil

1. Preheat the oven to 160°C (gas 3) and line a baking tray with baking paper.

2. Whisk the egg whites and rice malt syrup together. Stir in the coconut, quinoa and salt and place in the fridge for 1 hour. Scoop the quinoa mixture into 'blobs' and arrange on the prepared baking tray. Use your fingers to mould the blobs into small domes.

3. Bake for 15 minutes until golden brown. Once cooked, remove from the oven and allow to cool. Place the macaroons in the fridge for 1 hour to set hard.

4. Meanwhile, melt the chocolate and coconut oil, stirring together until combined. Remove the macaroons from the fridge and drizzle the chocolate over them, or dip the tips. Place back onto the baking tray and into the fridge for the chocolate to set – about 10 minutes.

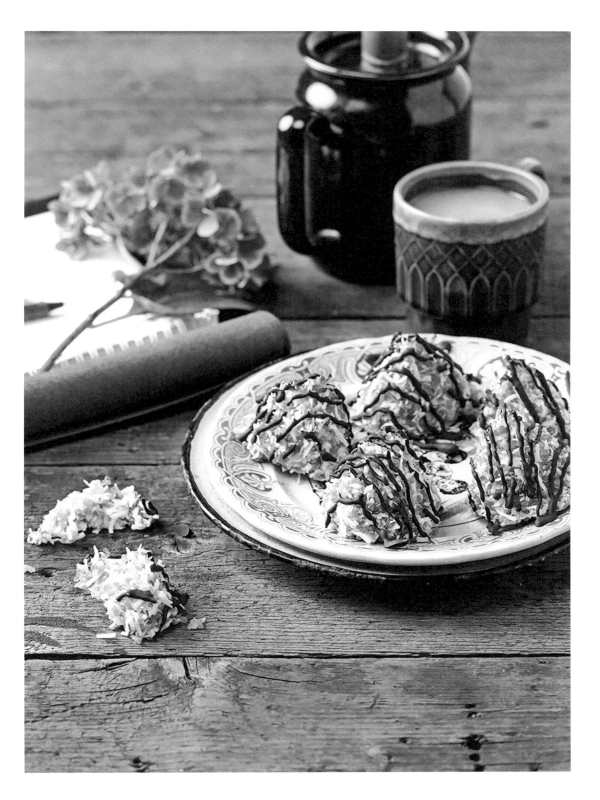

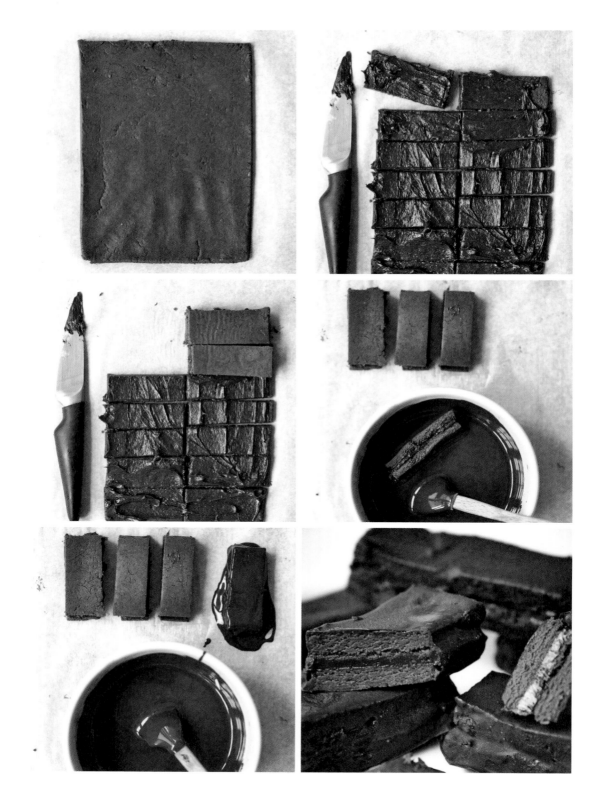

FUDGY DOUBLE CHOC BISCUITS

Tim Tams are an Australian icon. We force-feed them to overseas friends and celebrities are often made to eat them on our talk shows. The best way to enjoy these is dipped in a cup of tea. Don't mind if the biscuit crumbles. That's the best bit!

MAKES 8

PREPARATION TIME
1 hour

COOKING TIME
10 minutes

BISCUIT

1 cup (115 g) gluten-free flour + extra for dusting

½ tablespoon granulated stevia

⅓ cup (30 g) raw cacao powder

75 g cold butter, diced

¼ cup (60 ml) milk

FILLING

⅓ cup (75 ml) Chocolate Buttercream Frosting (see page 159)

CHOCOLATE COATING

100 g dark chocolate (85% cocoa), chopped into small even-sized pieces

1. Preheat the oven to 180°C (gas 4) and line a baking tray with baking paper. In a food processor or a mixing bowl combine all of the biscuit ingredients to form a dough. Transfer the dough to a lightly floured surface and knead until smooth. Roll dough out between two sheets of baking paper into a rectangle shape (about 5-mm thick).

2. Transfer to the tray and cut into 16 smaller rectangles and bake for 10 minutes. Once cooled, spread a thin layer of the filling over each biscuit.

3. Sandwich two biscuits on top of each other and press down lightly. Sit them in the fridge while you make the coating.

4. Melt the chocolate over a double boiler or in the microwave until smooth.

5. Dip each biscuit sandwich in the melted chocolate and sit them on baking paper. Place in the fridge to set before serving.

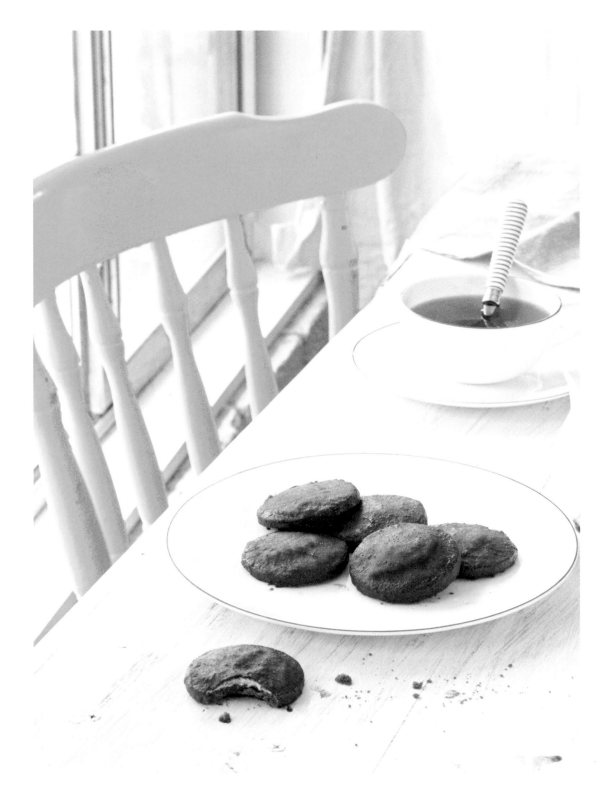

MINT SLICE

MAKES 18

PREPARATION TIME
40 minutes

COOKING TIME
15 minutes

BISCUITS

1 cup (115 g) gluten-free flour + extra for dusting

½ tablespoon granulated stevia or 2 tablespoons rice malt syrup

⅓ cup (30 g) raw cacao powder

75 g cold unsalted butter, diced

¼ cup (60 ml) milk

PEPPERMINT CREAM FILLING

⅓ cup (75 ml) Coconut Butter (see page 156), softened

peppermint oil (or essence), to taste

RAW CHOCOLATE COATING

6 tablespoons raw cacao powder

¼ cup (60 ml) rice malt syrup

⅓ cup (70 g) coconut oil, melted

1. To make the biscuits, preheat the oven to 180°C (gas 4) and line a baking tray with baking paper. Combine the flour, stevia and cacao in a large bowl or food processor. Add the diced butter and process or rub together with your fingers until the mixture resembles fine breadcrumbs.

2. Add the milk and rice malt syrup and mix to form a dough. Transfer to a lightly floured surface and knead for another minute or so, until the dough is nice and smooth.

3. Flatten the dough and place between two sheets of non-stick baking paper. Using a rolling pin, roll the dough out until it's about 3-mm thick. Cut out rounds and transfer to the prepared tray. Reroll the scraps and repeat the process.

4. Prick each biscuit with a fork a few times. Bake for 10 minutes then transfer to a wire rack to cool.

5. To make the filling, combine the Coconut Butter with a few drops of peppermint essence.

6. Spread ¾ of a teaspoon of the mixture onto the centre of each biscuit and leave to set in the fridge.

7. Set out a wire rack with baking paper underneath.

8. To make the chocolate coating, combine the cacao, rice malt syrup and melted coconut oil and mix well.

9. Dip the biscuits in the chocolate until coated and place on the wire rack in the fridge to set. Repeat process if you want to double coat biscuits.

TRICKY TIP

Keep mint slices in the fridge to avoid them melting. Eat within three days.

COCONUT ROUGHS

These could not be simpler to make and they taste like the real deal! Here at IQS HQ, we've been known to whip up a batch after lunch to satiate any sweet cravings.

MAKES 12

PREPARATION TIME
30 minutes

COOKING TIME
5 minutes

½ cup (100 g) coconut oil

2 tablespoons rice malt syrup

¼ cup (25 g) raw cacao powder

pinch of sea salt

½ cup (50 g) desiccated coconut

1.   Line a 12-cup muffin tray with paper cases.

2.   Melt the coconut oil and rice malt syrup in a microwave-safe bowl, stirring to combine. Add the cacao, salt and coconut and stir again.

3.   Spoon the mixture evenly into the lined muffin tray and flatten with a spoon. Set in the freezer before serving.

SHOW STOPPERS

*Whip up one of these for a special occasion
and hear the crowd gasp and exclaim,
'that can't be sugar-free!'*

ZOE'S FAVOURITE CARAMEL DRIZZLE CAKE

Upon eating this devilishly rich cake, Zoe (former CEO of IQS) announced that this was her favourite and could we not let her forget it. So, here you go, Zoe. A special cake dedicated to you!

SERVES 14

PREPARATION TIME
10 minutes

COOKING TIME
40 minutes

2 cups (200 g) almond meal

1 cup (100 g) desiccated coconut

½ cup (50 g) raw cacao powder

2 teaspoons baking powder

4 eggs, whisked

½ cup (115 g) butter, melted

¼ cup (60 ml) rice malt syrup

½ cup (120 ml) Gooey Caramel Sauce (see page 162)

1. Preheat oven to 180°C (gas 4) and line a 20 cm spring-form cake tin.

2. In a large bowl combine all of the ingredients except for the caramel sauce. Mix well to form a smooth batter. Spoon mixture into pre-lined baking tin.

3. Cook for 35–40 minutes until a skewer comes out clean when inserted.

4. Allow cake to cool for 5 minutes before removing from the tin.

5. Pour caramel sauce over the cake and serve immediately.

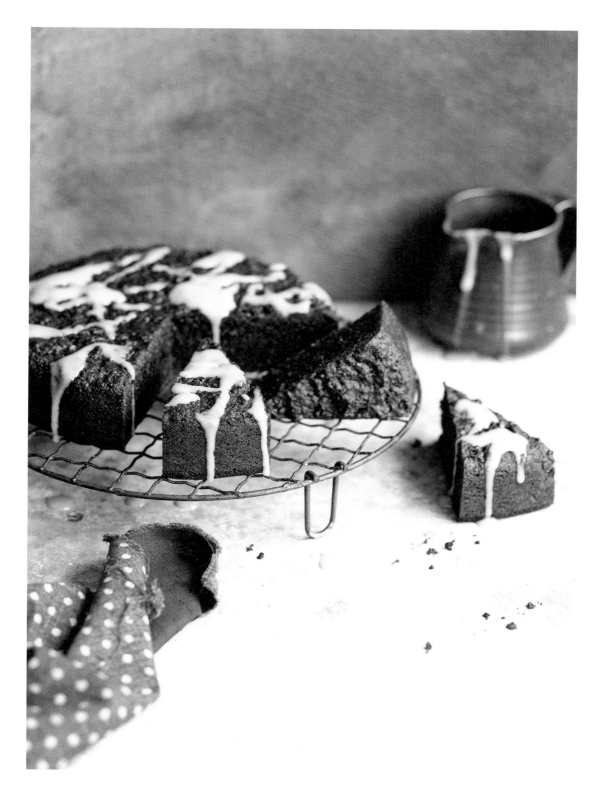

CHOCOLATE AVOCADO TART

This tart is packed with unsuspecting, nutritious ingredients! Yep, in order to achieve a beautiful creamy texture we use avocados. Before you turn your nose up, know this: you can't taste them ... we promise!

SERVES 12

PREPARATION TIME
3 hours

COOKING TIME
10 minutes

BASE

coconut oil, butter or ghee, for greasing

2 cups (200 g) almond meal

50 g butter, melted

2 tablespoons rice malt syrup

FILLING

2 ripe avocados

½ cup (120 ml) coconut cream, chilled so that it's firm

¼ cup (25 g) raw cacao powder

1 tablespoon chia seeds

2 teaspoons rice malt syrup

1 teaspoon vanilla powder or extract, optional

½ teaspoon ground cinnamon

pinch of sea salt

TOPPING

2 cups (300 g) fresh berries (any type you like)

1. Preheat oven to 180°C (gas 4) and grease a round 22 cm spring-form tart tin.

2. In a medium bowl, combine almond meal, butter and rice malt syrup together and then press firmly into cake tin.

3. Bake for 10 minutes and then remove from oven and set aside to cool.

4. In a blender combine all the filling ingredients until smooth. Spoon into cooled tart shell and refrigerate for at least 3 hours. To serve, arrange berries on top.

CHOC-CARAMEL-CHUNK AND PEANUT BUTTER 'CHEESECAKE'

An extract from I Quit Sugar for Life *by Sarah Wilson.*

Sarah says

" I wanted to create a party-stopping, ultra indulgence inciting the most hardened sweet tooth to cry out, "I can't believe THAT'S not sugar." This was the result. Be warned: it is super-rich (albeit dense in nutrients) and sweet (albeit via the coco-nuttiness). So it should be treated as... a treat, okay? (Take note of the servings.) "

SERVES 14

PREPARATION TIME
Overnight + 1 hour

COOKING TIME
20 minutes

CRUST

4½ cups (500 g) pecans

2 tablespoons raw cacao powder

1½ tablespoons coconut oil, melted

1 tablespoon vanilla powder
or extract, optional

1½ tablespoons rice malt syrup

CARAMEL SAUCE

100 g butter, chopped

¼ cup (60 ml) rice malt syrup

½ cup (120 ml) coconut cream

PRALINE

¼ cup (60 ml) rice malt syrup

1 cup (225 g) peanuts or macadamias,
or both, roughly chopped

ICE CREAM FILLING

3 cups (450 g) raw unsalted cashews

1¼ cups (300 ml) coconut cream

3 small avocados

⅓ cup (30 g) raw cacao powder

1½ teaspoons sea salt

1½ tablespoons granulated stevia

¾ teaspoon ground cinnamon

1½ cups (340 g) natural, sugar-free and
salt-free crunchy peanut butter

1½ tablespoons cacao nibs

CHOCOLATE SAUCE

¼ cup (50 g) coconut oil

1½ tablespoons rice malt syrup

1½ tablespoons raw cacao powder

small pinch of sea salt

1 tablespoon coconut cream

CONTINUED ON NEXT PAGE >

CHOC-CARAMEL-CHUNK AND PEANUT BUTTER 'CHEESECAKE'

(CONTINUED)

1. Line the bottom and sides of a round 23 cm spring-form tin with baking paper then start by making the crust.

2. Pulse the pecans in a food processor until roughly chopped. Add the remaining ingredients and process until the mixture has a moist, crumbly consistency. Spoon the mixture into the prepared tin and spread evenly around the base and 5 cm up the sides. Place in the fridge or freezer to set.

3. To make the caramel sauce, melt the butter with the rice malt syrup in a small saucepan over high heat. Bring to the boil, and then reduce the heat to medium so that the mixture keeps bubbling for about 8–10 minutes – do not stir or the caramel will split.

4. Cook for a further 4 minutes or until the caramel has turned golden and appears gooey when dripping off the back of a spoon. Remove from the heat and add the coconut cream, stirring gently. Transfer to a bowl and allow to cool.

5. To make the praline, preheat the grill and line a baking tray with baking paper. Warm the syrup gently, then mix with the nuts and transfer to the prepared tray. Grill for 5 minutes or until most of the water has evaporated and the syrup has turned golden and crystallised around the nuts.

6. Remove from the grill and cool, and then smash the praline into smaller pieces. Reserve 8 tablespoons for the topping, and keep the rest for the ice cream filling.

7. To make the filling, pulse the cashews with ½ cup (120 ml) of the coconut cream in a food processor until the mixture is smooth and buttery. Transfer to a large bowl and set aside.

8. Again using the food processor, pulse the avocados with the remaining coconut cream, cacao, salt and stevia until smooth. Add the cashew mixture, and then add the cinnamon, peanut butter, cacao nibs and praline. Stir well to combine.

9. Spoon about half of the filling mixture over the crust in the spring-form tin and spread right to the edges of the crust. Freeze for 5–10 minutes, then drizzle over half the caramel sauce. Freeze for another 5–10 minutes then add the remaining ice cream mixture.

10. Freeze for a further 5–10 minutes, then add the remaining caramel sauce and freeze the assembled cake for at least 6 hours, or overnight.

11. To make the chocolate sauce, place the coconut oil and rice malt syrup in a small saucepan and melt together over low heat. Remove from the heat and whisk through the cacao powder and salt until thoroughly combined, with no lumps.

12. Leave to cool for 5 minutes, then whisk through the coconut cream until smooth. (This sauce will thicken as it cools and can be reheated to make it runnier.) If the mixture makes more sauce than you need, just pour it into moulds and make some chocolates.

13. To serve, remove the cake from the freezer and transfer from the tin to a serving plate. Arrange the reserved praline around the edge of the plate and drizzle over the chocolate sauce. Allow to stand for 5 minutes before serving.

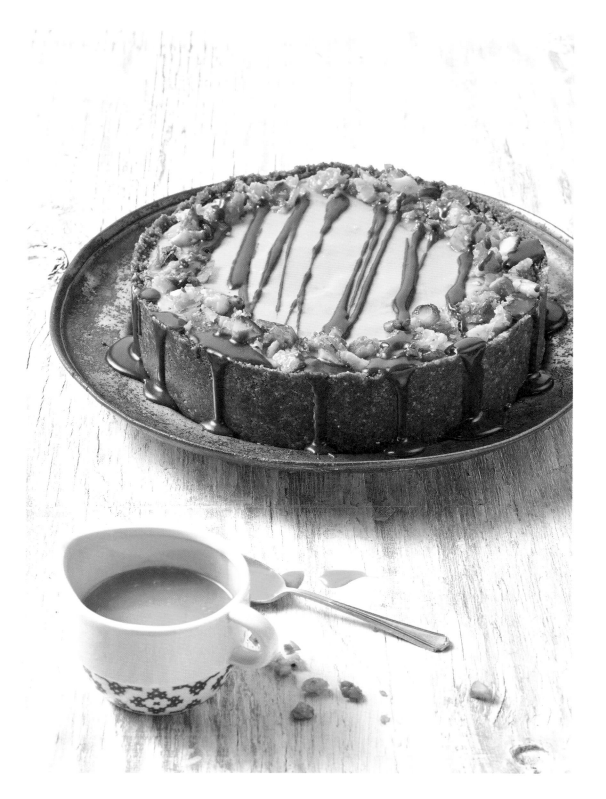

RAW CHOCOLATE 'N' SNEAKY BERRY 'CHEESECAKE'

The trick with serving this tasty vegan cake is getting it to room temperature. It'll taste like creamy mousse and wow your guests. The hidden berries will be a pleasant surprise, too.

SERVES 14

PREPARATION TIME
2 hours 15 minutes

CRUST

2 cups (225 g) pecans

¼ cup (25 g) raw cacao powder

¼ cup (60 ml) rice malt syrup

2 tablespoons coconut oil, melted

pinch of sea salt

FILLING

2½ cups (375 g) pre-soaked cashews

½ cup (50 g) raw cacao powder

¼ cup (60 ml) rice malt syrup

¼ cup (50 g) coconut oil

1 teaspoon vanilla powder

pinch of sea salt

1–2 tablespoons coconut milk (or milk of your choice)

½ cup (60 g) frozen raspberries

hazelnuts, to serve

TO MAKE THE CRUST

1. Line the base of a round spring-form cake tin with baking paper.

2. Process pecans in a food processor until chunky crumbs form. Add remaining ingredients and process until just combined.

3. Pour mixture into the prepared tin. Press into base to cover evenly and form a crust. Place in freezer to set.

TO MAKE THE FILLING

1. Process cashews until fine crumbs form. Add remaining ingredients except milk and raspberries. Process until mixture turns into a smooth and creamy batter.

2. Add milk as necessary to smooth out mixture. Once smooth, fold through raspberries and pour mixture over base in tin.

3. Refrigerate for at least 2 hours. Sprinkle with hazelnuts before serving.

TRICKY TIP

This cake can be stored in the freezer. Always allow it to thaw before serving. If it's too frozen it won't have the luscious, cheesecake-like texture you're after.

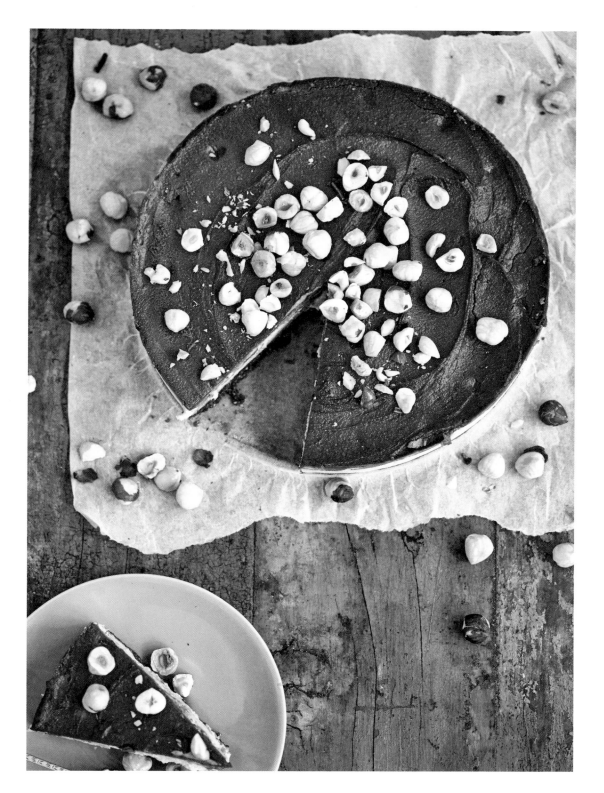

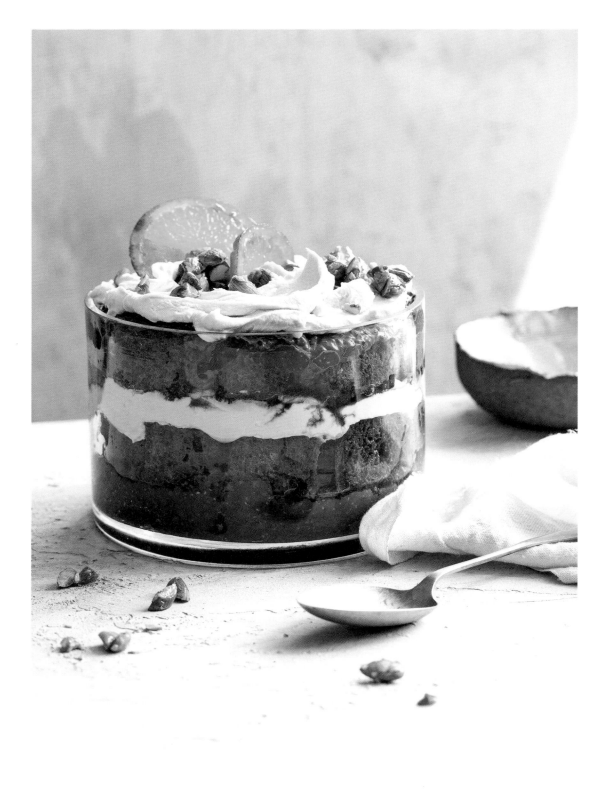

LEFTOVERS CHOC-ORANGE TIRAMISU WITH CANDIED ALMONDS

This is a sure-fire crowd pleaser. The combination of rich mousse, cream, coffee and a chocolate loaf makes these tiramisus super rich and wonderfully satisfying. Did we mention the candied nuts on top?

SERVES 6–8

PREPARATION TIME
15 minutes

COOKING TIME
6 minutes

1 cup (135 g) almonds, chopped

2½ tablespoons rice malt syrup

½ Chocolate Courgette Loaf
(see page 26), cut into 3-cm cubes

2 tablespoons instant coffee
granules

2 tablespoons boiling water

1 cup (250 ml) Vegan Jaffa Joy Mousse
(see page 56)

1½ cups (375 ml) Whipped Coconut
Cream (see page 158)

1. Preheat the oven to 180°C (gas 4). Spread the almonds on a lined baking tray, drizzle with 2 teaspoons of the rice malt syrup and toast for about 6 minutes, until golden and fragrant. Set aside.

2. Place loaf cubes in a large bowl. In a small bowl, combine instant coffee with hot water and remaining rice malt syrup until dissolved. Pour this mixture over the loaf cubes. Stir gently and set aside for 5 minutes.

3. To assemble, spoon a layer of Vegan Mousse at the base of each jar or glass, then a layer of loaf cubes and then a layer of coconut cream. Repeat process, finishing with the cream on top. Sprinkle candied nuts over the top to serve.

TRICKY TIP

To add flavour allow the loaf cubes to sit in the coffee mixture overnight before assembling.

SERVING SUGGESTION

For a burst of extra flavour, add slices of oranges that have been drizzled with rice malt syrup and quickly pan fried.

SIMPLE CHOCOLATE COCONUT MILK ICE CREAM

This four-ingredient ice cream will knock your guests off their seat when you tell them it's fructose-free! Serve with some Ice Magic to make this treat the ultimate party food.

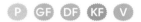

SERVES 4

PREPARATION TIME
5 hours 5 minutes

1 x 400 ml can full-fat coconut milk

⅓ cup (30 g) raw cacao powder

1 tablespoon rice malt syrup

½ teaspoon vanilla powder

Ice Magic (see page 161), to serve

1. Mix all of the ingredients together in a blender, or use a stick blender, until smooth and creamy. Pour into a freezer-safe container (a lunch box will do).

2. Place in the freezer and leave for 5 hours. Alternatively, you can use an ice cream maker, if you have one.

3. Once frozen, serve with Ice Magic.

TRICKY TIP

The ice cream may become a little too firm in the freezer if left for too long. If so, allow to thaw on your worktop for a few minutes before serving.

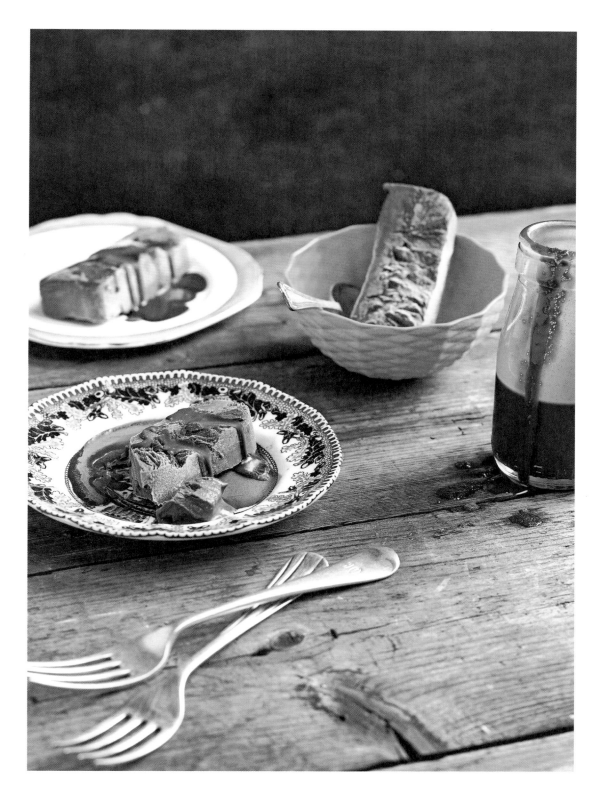

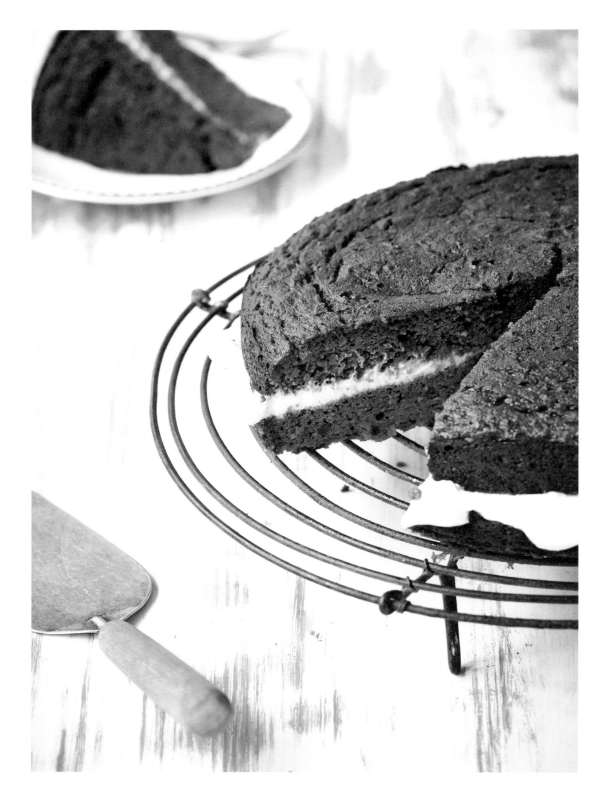

CHOCOLATE RED VELVET CAKE WITH CREAM CHEESE FROSTING

Not only is this cake fantastically vibrant when served up, it's also jam-packed with beetroot. Beets are great for reducing inflammation and supporting the body through detoxification. The addition of beets also gives this cake a moist and fluffy texture without sacrificing flavour.

SERVES 12

PREPARATION TIME
15 minutes

COOKING TIME
45 minutes

⅓ cup (30 g) raw cacao powder

½ cup (60 g) coconut flour

2 teaspoons baking powder

pinch of sea salt

2 teaspoons vanilla extract

8 eggs, whisked

⅓ cup (75 ml) rice malt syrup

½ cup (100 g) coconut oil, melted

2 cups (300 g) grated beetroot

1 cup (250 g) Cream Cheese Frosting (see page 159), to serve

1. Line a round spring-form cake tin with baking paper and preheat the oven to 180°C (gas 4). Add all dry ingredients into a mixing bowl and mix until combined.

2. In a separate bowl, whisk together the wet ingredients. Add in the dry ingredients and fold through the grated beetroot.

3. Pour mixture into the tin and bake for 40–45 minutes or until a skewer comes out clean when inserted in the middle. Remove cake from the oven and set aside to cool completely.

4. Once cool, carefully remove cake from the tin and slice in half width ways with a sharp knife.

5. Spread the bottom layer of the cake with frosting and place the other layer carefully on top. Serve.

NUT-ELLA CHEESECAKE

Homemade Choc Hazelnut Spread and cheesecake. Need we say more?

SERVES 16

PREPARATION TIME
3 hours

COOKING TIME
10 minutes

BASE

60 g butter, melted

2 cups (200 g) almond meal

½ teaspoon sea salt

NUT-ELLA FILLING

500 g cream cheese

2 tablespoons coconut milk

2 tablespoons rice malt syrup

1½ cups (375 ml) Choc Hazelnut Spread (see page 165)

2 tablespoons raw cacao powder

40 g dark chocolate (85% cocoa), chopped into even-sized pieces, to serve

¼ cup (30 g) hazelnuts, roughly chopped + extra to serve

1. Preheat the oven to 180°C (gas 4) and line a round 22 cm spring-form cake tin with baking paper. To make the base, combine the butter, almond meal and salt in a bowl. Mix well. The more you work the mixture the better it will turn out.

2. Press the mixture into the bottom of the tin and bake for 10 minutes until golden. Remove from the oven and allow to cool fully.

3. Meanwhile combine all the filling ingredients in a blender until well mixed. Pour mixture over the base and sit in the fridge for at least 3 hours.

4. Melt the chocolate in the microwave or over a double boiler. To serve, turn cheesecake out of the tin, top with hazelnuts and drizzle with chocolate.

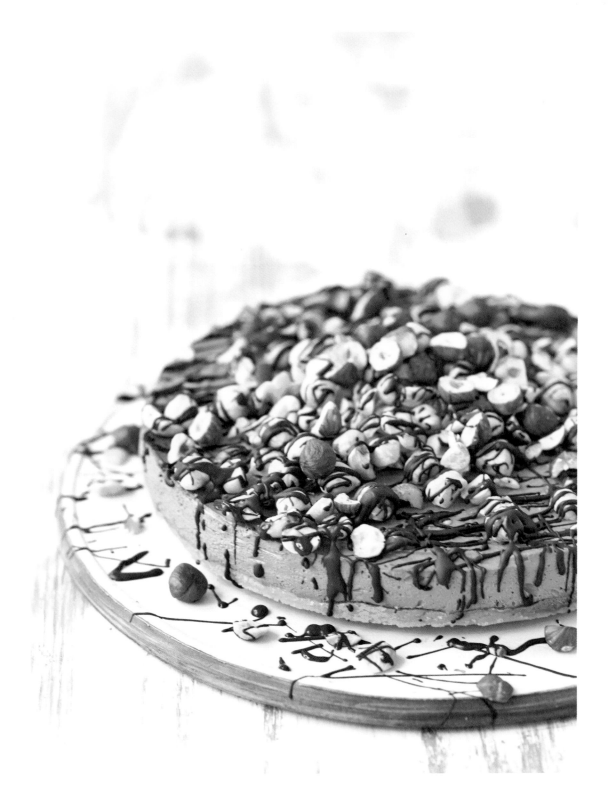

COURGETTE MUD CAKE WITH CHOCOLATE GANACHE AND SALTED CARAMEL POPCORN

This cake is a show stopper and literally left Sarah and the IQS Team lost for words. Make this cake if you want to wow your guests for a special occasion ... Oh yeah, we snuck in some veggies too.

A caveat: *This cake should always be enjoyed in moderation.*

SERVES 12

PREPARATION TIME
10 minutes

COOKING TIME
40 minutes

CHOCOLATE CAKE

½ cup (50 g) raw cacao powder

½ cup (60 g) coconut flour

1 tablespoon baking powder

2 teaspoons vanilla powder or extract, optional

pinch of sea salt

8 eggs, whisked

¼ cup (60 ml) rice malt syrup

½ cup (100 g) coconut oil (or butter), melted

2 cups (450 g) courgette, grated and squeezed of any excess moisture

1 cup (250 ml) Chocolate Buttercream Frosting (see page 159)

100 g dark chocolate (85% cocoa), chopped into even-sized pieces (or 1 cup/250 ml Basic Raw Chocolate, see page 13)

SALTED CARAMEL POPCORN

2 cups (25 g) air-popped popcorn

⅓ cup (75 ml) Gooey Caramel Sauce (see page 162)

1. Preheat the oven to 180°C (gas 4) and line a round 22 cm spring-form cake tin with baking paper. Combine all the chocolate cake ingredients except for the Chocolate Buttercream and dark chocolate in a large bowl until a smooth batter forms.

2. Pour batter into the tin and cook for 40 minutes or until the top is firm to the touch and a skewer comes out clean when inserted in centre of cake. Set cake aside to cool completely.

3. Meanwhile make the Salted Caramel Popcorn by combining the popcorn and Gooey Caramel Sauce in a bowl. Sit in the fridge to set.

4. Once cooled, slice the cake in half. Spread the base with Chocolate Buttercream Frosting. Place the top layer carefully back on top. Melt chocolate over a double boiler or in the microwave until smooth. Pour over the cake. Top with popcorn and serve.

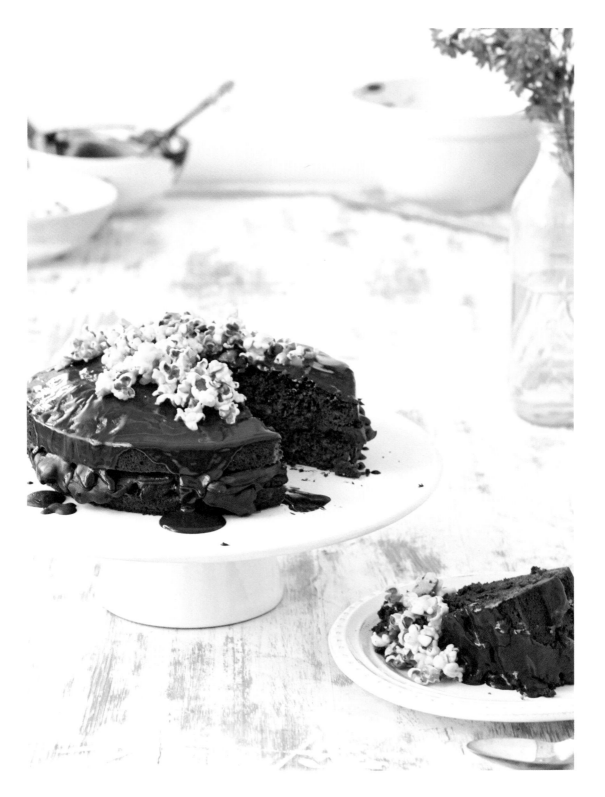

MOCHA AND HAZELNUT LAYER CAKE

Recipe by Zainab of Lagallette.com
This is a gorgeous contributor recipe from Lagallette.com. We couldn't believe
a 16-year-old was capable of developing such a drool-worthy cake! It certainly
stopped us in our tracks.

SERVES 14

PREPARATION TIME
1 hour 15 minutes

COOKING TIME
25 minutes

CAKE

coconut oil, butter or ghee, for greasing

½ cup (60 g) coconut flour (or flour of your choice)

½ cup (50 g) raw cacao powder

2 teaspoons baking powder

1 teaspoon bicarbonate of soda

8 eggs

¼ cup (60 ml) rice malt syrup

½ cup (100 g) coconut oil, melted

1 teaspoon vanilla powder or extract, optional

dark chocolate (85% cocoa), flaked, to decorate

roasted hazelnuts, roughly chopped, to decorate

FROSTING

3 cups (750 ml) Whipped Coconut Cream (see page 158)

1 tablespoon espresso, cold

¼ cup (25 g) raw cacao powder

2 tablespoons coconut oil, softened

1 tablespoon rice malt syrup

1. Preheat the oven to 180°C (gas 4). Grease two round 20 cm cake tins and line the bases with baking paper. Set aside.

2. Sift the flour, cacao, baking powder and bicarbonate of soda into a large bowl.

3. Add the eggs, rice malt syrup, melted coconut oil and vanilla and whisk until smooth.

4. Divide the batter between the prepared tins and rest for 5 minutes.

5. Bake for 20–25 minutes or until a skewer inserted into the middle of the cake comes out clean. Cool completely.

6. Whisk together the Whipped Coconut Cream, espresso, cacao, coconut oil and rice malt syrup until combined.

7. Place one cake round on a cake board or plate. Spread half the frosting onto the cake, smoothing out but leaving a 2 cm gap around the edge.

8. Sprinkle with flaked chocolate and hazelnuts. Place on the second cake. Spread on the remaining frosting and sprinkle with the remaining chocolate and hazelnuts.

9. Refrigerate for 1 hour before serving.

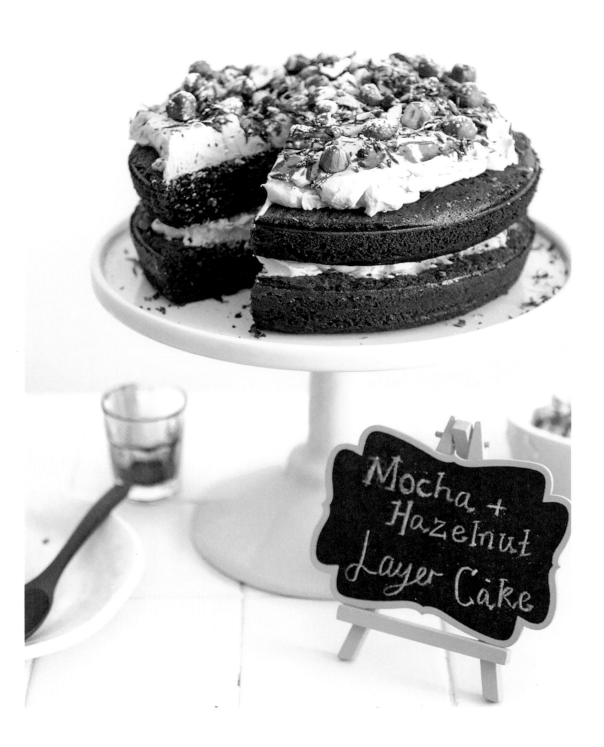

Mocha + Hazelnut Layer Cake

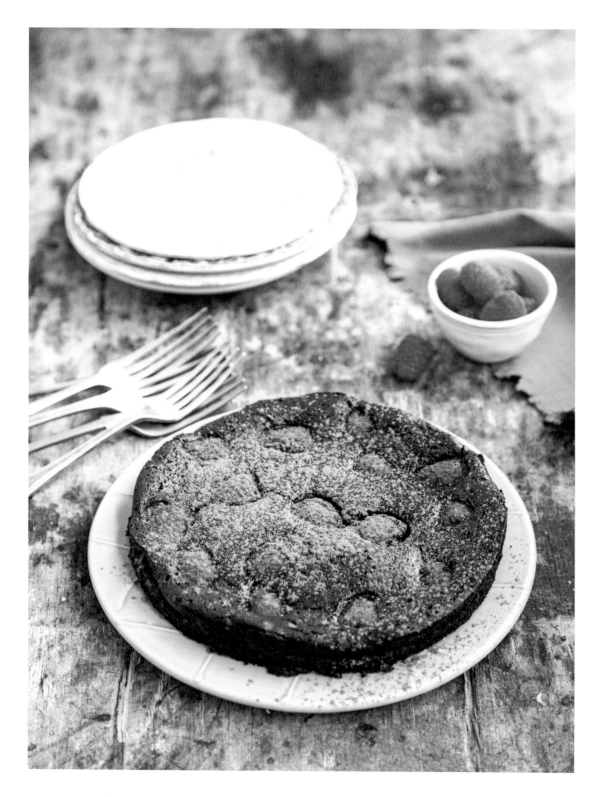

FLOURLESS BERRY CHOCOLATE CAKE

Even if you're not gluten intolerant this recipe will wow your mates. It tastes like fudge and cake combined. The addition of berries helps to cut through the richness of this moreish treat.

SERVES 14

PREPARATION TIME
10 minutes

COOKING TIME
30 minutes

coconut oil, butter or ghee, for greasing

½ cup (100 g) coconut oil

100 g dark chocolate (85% cocoa), chopped into even-sized pieces

¼ cup (25 g) raw cacao powder + extra for dusting, optional

1 teaspoon ground cinnamon

pinch of sea salt

¼ cup (60 ml) rice malt syrup

3 eggs, whisked

1 punnet fresh raspberries

1. Grease a round 20 cm spring-form tin generously. Preheat the oven to 200°C (gas 6).

2. Melt coconut oil in the microwave. Pour oil over chocolate chunks in a separate bowl and stir until smooth and combined.

3. Add the cacao, cinnamon, salt, rice malt syrup and eggs and whisk until a smooth batter forms. Gently stir through raspberries, reserving a few.

4. Pour batter into the greased tin and level out with the back of a spoon or spatula. Top with extra raspberries.

5. Bake for 25 minutes, until the centre looks just firm. Set aside to cool before removing from the tin. Dust with cacao, if you like.

CHOCOLATE PEANUT BUTTER CRACKLES

Seven ingredients, one pot, 4½ minutes, some time in the fridge, and you're done. An extract from I Quit Sugar: Simplicious *by Sarah Wilson.*

MAKES 18

PREPARATION TIME
2 hours 10 minutes

COOKING TIME
5 minutes

¾ cup (150 g) coconut oil

2 tablespoons rice malt syrup

¼ cup (25 g) raw cacao powder

½ cup (115 g) crunchy natural peanut butter

½ cup (40 g) desiccated coconut

½ cup (85 g) 'activated groaties' (activated buckwheat groats)

1½ cups (40 g) puffed quinoa or puffed rice

1. Line two cupcake trays or muffin tins with 18 paper cases.

2. Gently heat the coconut oil in a saucepan over a low–medium heat. Remove from the heat and stir in the rice malt syrup. Add the cacao and peanut butter and stir to combine. Add the coconut, groaties and puffed quinoa or rice and mix well. Spoon the mixture into the prepared trays. Refrigerate for 2 hours to completely set, then serve. Store leftovers in a sealed container in the fridge for up to 2 weeks.

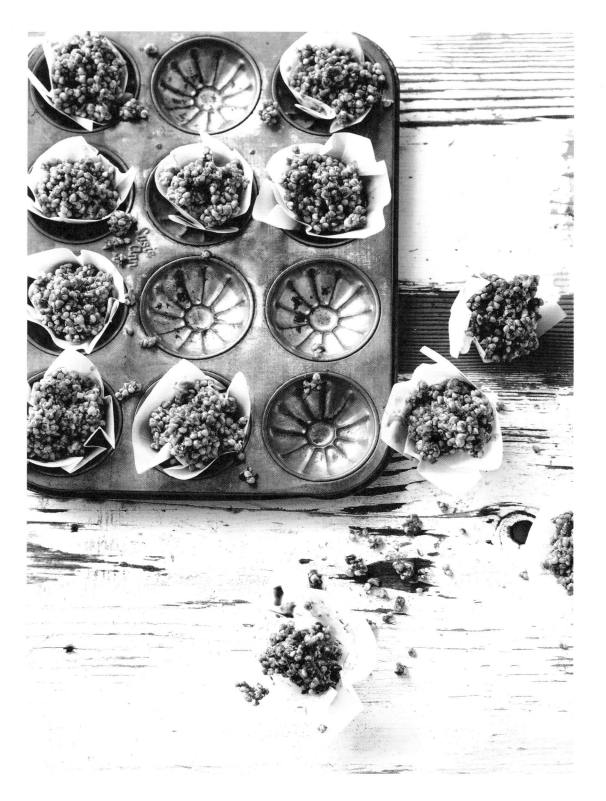

SELF-SAUCING PUDDING

Recipe by Alice Nicholls of thewholedaily.com.au

SERVES 4–6

PREPARATION TIME
15 minutes

COOKING TIME
30 minutes

PUDDING

1 cup (120 g) buckwheat flour

⅔ cup (150 ml) almond milk (or milk of your choice)

⅓ cup (30 g) raw cacao powder

⅓ cup (70 g) coconut oil or ⅓ cup (75 ml) olive oil

¼ cup (60 ml) rice malt syrup

1 egg, lightly beaten

½ teaspoon baking powder

¼ teaspoon bicarbonate of soda

1 teaspoon apple cider vinegar

Whipped Coconut Cream (see page 158), to serve, optional

CHOCOLATE SAUCE

¼ cup (25 g) raw cacao powder

1 tablespoon rice malt syrup

1¼ cups (300 ml) boiling water

1. Preheat the oven to 180°C (gas 4) and grease a round 20 cm baking dish or four ramekins.

2. Mix together pudding ingredients until combined into a batter.

3. Pour into baking dish or ramekins.

4. Mix together all the ingredients for chocolate sauce in a small bowl.

5. Using a large spoon or spatula so you don't damage the pudding batter, carefully pour the sauce over the back of the spoon or spatula into the baking dish over the batter. You don't want to break the mix up too much as it may end up with a sloppy texture – so just go slow. Note: the chocolate sauce will float on top and as the pudding cooks it sinks to the bottom of the baking dish.

6. Bake for 20–30 minutes depending on your dish size, until the centre of the pudding is firm. Remove from the oven and dish up with a dollop of cream or serve as is.

TRICKY TIP

It's worth placing a tray under the rack the baking dish is on to catch any sauce that may bubble over the side during cooking.

WHEN YOU'RE ASKED TO 'BRING A PLATE'

These recipes are perfect when you have to bring a sweet treat to an office meeting or a morning tea.

MOLTEN PEANUT BUTTER 'N' JELLY BROWNIES

These originated as peanut butter brownies. It wasn't until Sarah suggested the addition of 'jelly' that they became really special.

SERVES 24

PREPARATION TIME
10 minutes

COOKING TIME
20–25 minutes

coconut oil, butter or ghee, for greasing

1½ cups (150 g) almond meal

¼ cup (25 g) raw cacao powder

1 teaspoon baking powder

½ teaspoon sea salt

½ cup (115 g) unsalted butter, melted

¼ cup (60 ml) rice malt syrup

3 eggs, lightly whisked

⅓ cup (75 g) crunchy peanut butter

½ cup (60 g) raspberries, mashed with a fork

1. Preheat the oven to 160°C (gas 3). Line a 22 cm square brownie tin with baking paper.

2. In a large bowl combine all of the ingredients, except for the peanut butter and raspberries, until smooth.

3. Pour the batter into the lined cake tin. Dollop peanut butter into mixture and use a skewer or knife to create a swirl pattern. Repeat the process with mashed raspberries.

4. Cook for 20–25 minutes, checking at 15 minutes to ensure mixture is not burning. Brownies are cooked when top is slightly firm to the touch. You want them to be gooey so try not to overcook.

5. Allow brownies to cool for 10 minutes before removing from the pan and slicing.

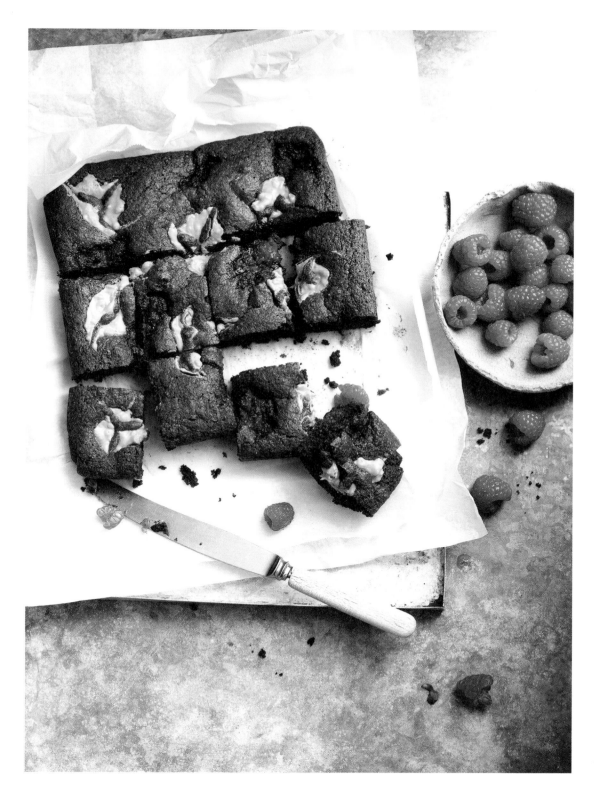

RUSTIC CHOCOLATEY PLUM FRANGIPANI TARTS

Nothing says summer like juicy stone fruit. You can make this recipe with any type you like.

MAKES 4

PREPARATION TIME
10 minutes

COOKING TIME
30 minutes

coconut, butter or oil, for greasing

90 g butter, softened

⅓ cup (75 ml) rice malt syrup

¼ cup (25 g) raw cacao powder

2 eggs

1 cup (100 g) almond meal

¼ cup (25 g) plain gluten-free flour

½ teaspoon gluten-free baking powder

1 teaspoon orange zest, finely grated

2 plums, halved, de-stoned and cut into thin wedges

1. Grease four small tart tins or a round 22 cm spring-form pie/quiche tin and preheat the oven to 160°C (gas 3).

2. Place the butter and rice malt syrup in a bowl or a food processor and mix until just combined. Add the cacao, eggs, almond meal, flour, baking powder and orange zest and process until combined.

3. Pour mixture into the tins and press the plum segments evenly around the edge of the mixture. Bake for 25–30 minutes or until cooked when tested with a skewer. Allow to cool in the tins before serving.

TRICKY TIP

This is delicious served with a drizzle of cream or a dollop of Whipped Coconut Cream (see page 158).

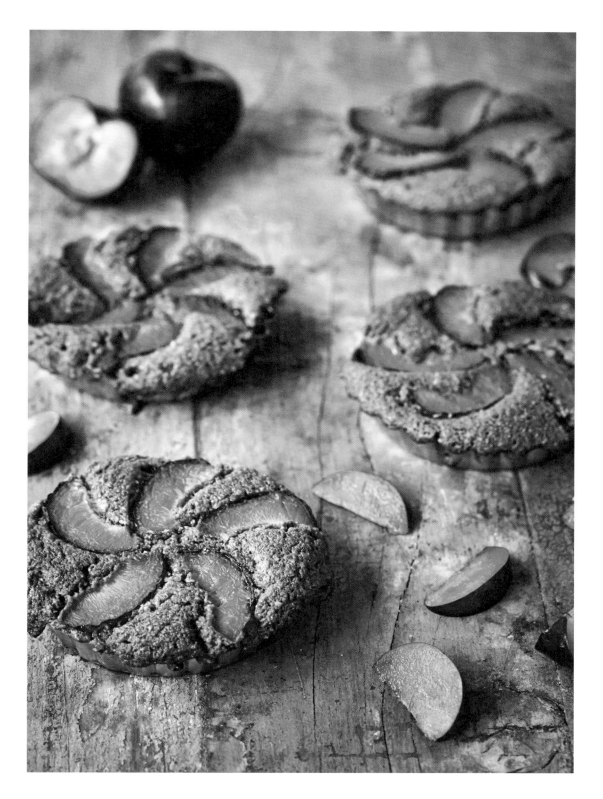

CHEESECAKE
SWIRL BROWNIES

*If you don't have a big sweet tooth then this recipe is great for you.
The cheese offsets the sweetness and you'll be very satisfied with
a small serving.*

MAKES 20

PREPARATION TIME
5 minutes

COOKING TIME
35 minutes

½ cup (100 g) coconut oil + extra,
for greasing

⅓ cup (75 ml) rice malt syrup

½ cup (50 g) raw cacao powder

1 cup (100 g) almond meal

½ cup (50 g) plain gluten-free flour
(or an extra cup/100 g of almond meal)

3 eggs

¼ cup (60 ml) sour cream

250 g cream cheese

½ teaspoon vanilla powder
or extract, optional

1. Preheat the oven to 180°C (gas 4). Grease a 22 cm square brownie tin and
   line with baking paper.

2. Melt coconut oil and rice malt syrup on stove and combine well. Remove
   from heat and cool for 5 minutes. Transfer to a bowl. Add cacao, almond
   meal and flour.

3. Lightly beat two eggs and add to cacao mixture. Combine well. Stir through
   sour cream.

4. Using electric beaters or a food processor beat cream cheese and vanilla
   until smooth. Add the remaining egg. Beat until just combined.

5. Spoon brownie mixture and cheese mixture in a checkerboard pattern
   across base of tin. Use the handle of a wooden spoon to form swirls
   in mixture.

6. Bake for 30 minutes or until a skewer inserted into the centre comes
   out clean.

CHOCOLATE DIPPED GINGERBREAD BISCUITS

Make up a big batch of these at Christmas time and give them as gifts to friends. They're also super yummy dunked in a morning coffee.

MAKES 25

PREPARATION TIME
2 hours 10 minutes

COOKING TIME
15 minutes

2½ cups (250 g) almond meal

¼ cup (30 g) coconut flour

1 teaspoon ground cinnamon

1 tablespoon ground ginger

2 pinches of ground cloves

½ teaspoon sea salt

1 teaspoon baking powder

50 g butter, melted

½ cup (120 ml) rice malt syrup

1 tablespoon orange zest

1 teaspoon vanilla powder or extract, optional

1 egg

½ cup (120 ml) Basic Raw Chocolate (see page 13) or 60 g dark chocolate (85% cocoa), melted

1. Preheat the oven to 180°C (gas 4) and line two baking trays with baking paper.

2. Place almond meal, flour, spices, salt and baking powder in a food processor and pulse briefly. Add butter, rice malt syrup, orange zest, vanilla and egg. Pulse until dough forms a ball. Wrap in clingfilm and place in the fridge for at least 2 hours.

3. Roll dough between two sheets of baking paper until 1-cm thick. Cut into shapes with a cookie cutter and place on baking trays.

4. Bake for 10–15 minutes until biscuits have a light golden brown tinge around the edges. Remove from the oven and set aside to cool. Dip biscuits halfway in Basic Raw Chocolate and sit on baking trays in the fridge until chocolate goes hard.

GANACHE-FILLED BROWNIE BITES

This was a special recipe developed for people on the online I Quit Sugar 8-Week Programme. It was such a hit that we thought we'd share it with you.

MAKES 16–18

PREPARATION TIME
5 minutes

COOKING TIME
10 minutes

BISCUITS

¼ cup (25 g) almond meal

½ cup (60 g) coconut flour

pinch of sea salt

¼ teaspoon bicarbonate of soda

¼ cup (25 g) raw cacao powder
+ extra to serve, optional

¼ cup (50 g) coconut oil, melted

2 tablespoons rice malt syrup

1 egg

GANACHE

60 g dark chocolate (85% cocoa)

3 tablespoons coconut cream,
at room temperature

1. Preheat the oven to 180°C (gas 4). Line a baking tray with baking paper.

2. To make the biscuits, combine all dry ingredients in a small bowl. Place all wet ingredients in a large bowl and whisk to combine. Add dry ingredients and mix until well combined.

3. Take teaspoonful amounts and roll into balls in the palm of your hand. Place on baking paper and gently press flat (about 3mm thick) with the back of a large spoon. You should get 16–18 biscuits. Bake for 10 minutes or until just firm to touch. Remove from the oven and allow to cool.

4. To make the ganache, gently melt chocolate over a double boiler in a ceramic heatproof bowl. Watch carefully and remove from the heat to ensure the mixture doesn't seize (split). Allow to cool for 1–2 minutes before adding coconut cream. Stir using a plastic spatula until mixture is thick and turns into a silky ganache.

5. Spoon teaspoons of the ganache between two biscuits and press gently together. Sprinkle with extra cacao, if you like. Serve.

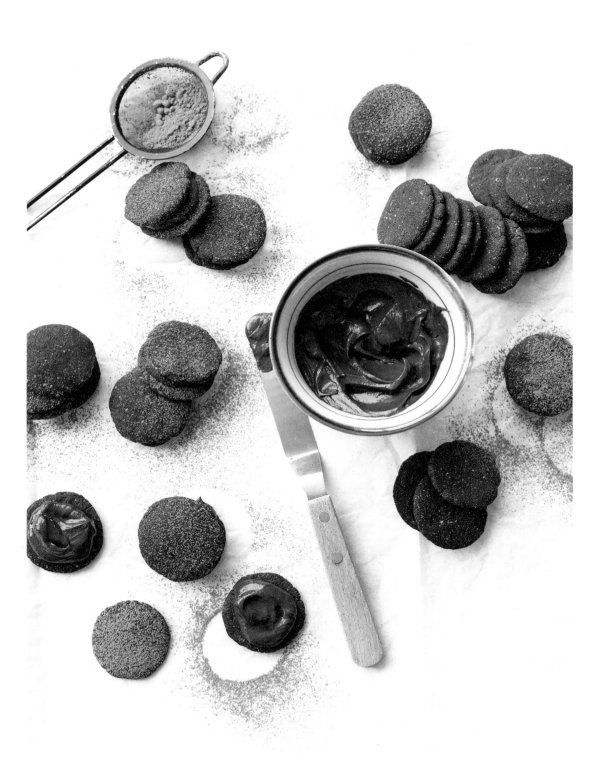

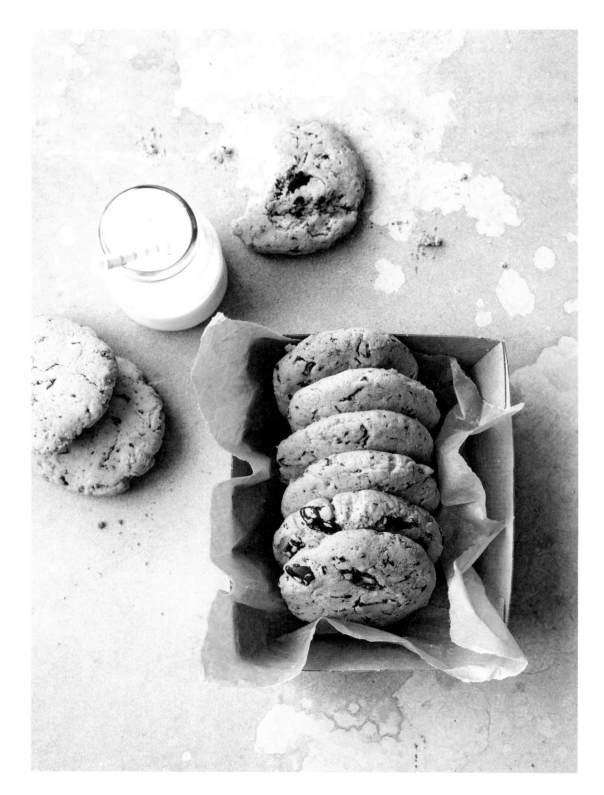

GLUTEN-FREE
CHOC-CHIP COOKIES

Ah, the humble choc-chip cookie. The buckwheat in these gives the biscuits an almost cake-like texture. We recommend you try them in your kids' lunch boxes. Yep, they're totally nut-free!

MAKES 12

PREPARATION TIME
5 minutes

COOKING TIME
20 minutes

1½ cups (175 g) buckwheat flour

1 teaspoon gluten-free baking powder

1 teaspoon vanilla powder or extract, optional

½ teaspoon sea salt

125 g unsalted butter, softened

⅓ cup (75 ml) rice malt syrup

1 egg

100 g dark chocolate (85% cocoa), coarsely chopped

1. Preheat the oven to 160°C (gas 3). Line two baking sheets with baking paper.

2. Combine flour, baking powder, vanilla powder, if using, and salt in a large bowl.

3. In a separate bowl beat butter, vanilla powder or extract, if using, and rice malt syrup until creamy. Add egg and beat until combined.

4. Add butter mixture to dry ingredients and combine with a wooden spoon. Fold through chocolate.

5. Spoon tablespoonfuls of the mixture into balls and place on the lined trays. Press down slightly.

6. Bake for 15–20 minutes until lightly golden. Transfer to a wire rack to cool. Store in an airtight container.

TRICKY TIP

If you want to reduce the fructose further, replace the dark chocolate with cacao nibs.

FLOURLESS
COURGETTE BROWNIE

We've smuggled some grated courgette into these decadent chocolate brownies.
They're incredibly rich, which is why we've kept the serving sizes small.

MAKES 12

PREPARATION TIME
10 minutes

COOKING TIME
35 minutes

coconut oil, for greasing

1 cup (225 g) almond butter

1 egg

½ teaspoon vanilla powder

1 tablespoon rice malt syrup

1 teaspoon ground cinnamon

¼ teaspoon ground nutmeg

1 teaspoon bicarbonate of soda

1 large courgette, grated and squeezed of any excess moisture

100 g dark chocolate (85–90% cocoa), roughly chopped

1. Preheat the oven to 180°C (gas 4) and grease a 22 cm square brownie tin.

2. Add all ingredients together in a large mixing bowl. Stir until combined and smooth. Scoop mixture into the prepared brownie tin and place in the oven. Bake for 35 minutes, or until a cocktail stick inserted in the centre comes out clean.

3. Remove from the oven and allow to cool slightly before slicing into small squares to serve. For an optional extra, drizzle with Basic Raw Chocolate (see page 13).

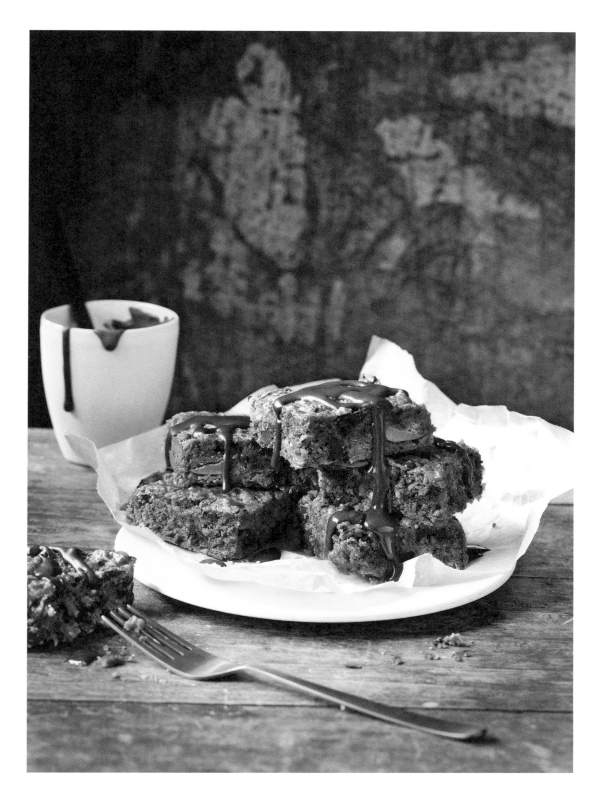

SWEET POTATO + MACADAMIA FUDGE BROWNIE

Adding sweet potato purée (or pumpkin if you like) to your brownie mixture gives the most incredible fudginess. Add some rich cacao and a little crunch from macadamias and you have the perfect nutrient-dense treat.

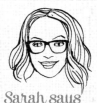

Sarah says

❝ I like my brownies a bit gooey. Test using a skewer; if it comes out a little moist, then you're good to go. If you like more of a cake texture, add on an extra 5–10 minutes of cooking time. Test using a skewer, and when it comes out clean it's ready. ❞

SERVES 14

PREPARATION TIME
10 minutes

COOKING TIME
30 minutes

coconut oil, for greasing

1½ cups (375 ml) Sweet Potato Purée (see page 166)

2 tablespoons rice malt syrup

90 g butter, softened

½ teaspoon vanilla powder

½ cup (50 g) self-raising flour

⅓ cup (30 g) raw cacao powder

¼ teaspoon baking powder

½ teaspoon cayenne pepper

pinch of sea salt

3 eggs, whisked

¾ cup (175 g) macadamia nuts, roughly chopped

50 g dark chocolate (85–90% cocoa), roughly chopped

1. Preheat the oven to 180°C (gas 4) and lightly grease a 22 cm x 35 cm brownie tin.

2. Add all the ingredients to a large mixing bowl. Stir together until a smooth batter is formed. Pour batter into prepared brownie tin and bake for 30 minutes.

3. Once cooked to your liking (see Sarah's note), remove from the oven and allow to cool slightly before slicing into small rectangles. This fudge tastes best when served cool.

RAW CHOCOLATE
STRAWBERRY BROWNIE

This one requires no baking. The recipe works better if you've chopped and frozen the strawberries in advance, but no drama if you only have fresh ones on hand.

(P) (GF) (DF) (V)

SERVES 14

PREPARATION TIME
1 hour 10 minutes

coconut oil, for greasing

⅓ cup (30 g) raw cacao powder

1 cup (100 g) almond meal

2 tablespoons chia seeds

1 cup (75 g) desiccated coconut

½ cup (120 ml) Pumpkin Purée
(see page 166)

1 teaspoon vanilla
powder, optional

2 tablespoons coconut
oil, melted

1 cup (150 g) frozen strawberries,
roughly chopped

2 cups (225 g) walnuts, roughly
chopped

1. Grease and line a 22 cm x 35 cm brownie tin.

2. Blend all ingredients except the strawberries and walnuts in a blender or use a stick blender. Stir in the strawberries and walnuts.

3. Pour mixture into the tin and place in the freezer for at least 1 hour.

4. Once set, remove and slice into squares to serve.

TRICKY TIP

Store these brownies in an airtight container in the fridge.

COURGETTE +
PEAR BROWNIE

Gluten-free, dairy-free and full of fibre, we've packed these decadent brownies with fruit and veg. The courgette gives the brownies a fudgy texture, while the pear provides a natural sweetness.

SERVES 12

PREPARATION TIME
10 minutes

COOKING TIME
20 minutes

¼ cup (50 g) coconut oil, melted + extra, for greasing

2 eggs

1 tablespoon rice malt syrup

1 teaspoon vanilla extract

1 small courgette, finely grated and squeezed of any excess moisture

1½ cups (150 g) almond meal

1 teaspoon baking powder

¼ cup (25 g) raw cacao powder

¼ teaspoon sea salt

1 pear

1. Preheat the oven to 180°C (gas 4) and grease a 22 cm square cake tin with coconut oil.

2. Add coconut oil, eggs, rice malt syrup and vanilla straight into the cake tin and combine with a rubber whisk to avoid ruining your tin. Add the grated courgette and whisk to combine.

3. Add the almond meal, baking powder, cacao and salt and stir until mixed together. Avoiding the pear seeds, roughly chop half of the pear into 2-cm cubes and fold through the brownie mixture.

4. Flatten the mixture in the tin and smooth with the back of a spoon or spatula. Thinly slice the remaining pear, removing seeds, and place fanned across the top of the brownie mixture. Bake for 20 minutes.

5. When cooked, remove from the oven and serve.

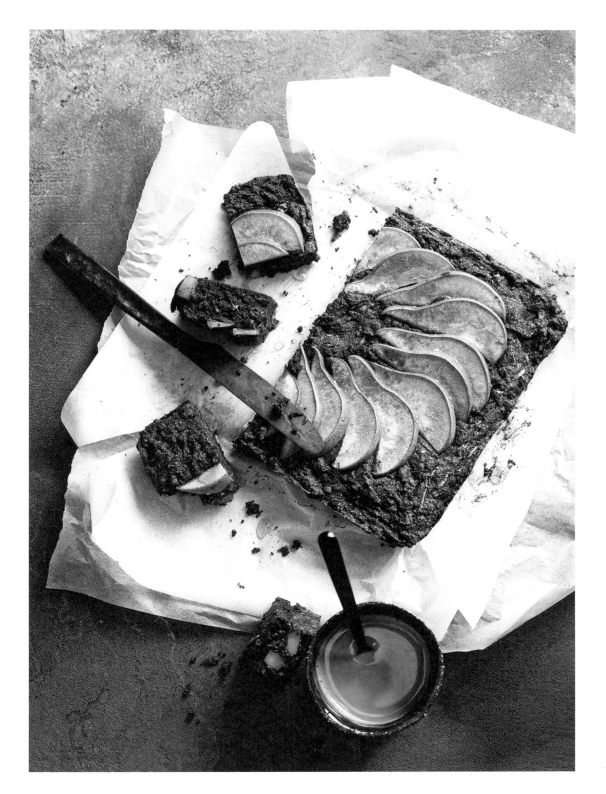

RASPBERRY RIPPLE

This is one of Sarah Wilson's most popular recipes in her first book I Quit Sugar, *and also on the* I Quit Sugar *website.*

SERVES 6

PREPARATION TIME
40 minutes

⅓ cup (50 g) frozen raspberries

⅓ cup (30 g) shredded coconut

⅓ cup (70 g) coconut oil

80 g salted butter

2 tablespoons raw cacao powder

2 tablespoons rice malt syrup

1. Line a dinner plate or baking tray with baking paper (a dinner plate is ideal as the slight indent creates a good shape). Scatter the berries and coconut on the plate or tray.

2. Melt the oil and butter together in a saucepan on low heat or in the microwave (the oil takes a little longer to melt, so add the butter a little after), then whisk in the cacao and the rice malt syrup.

3. Pour the chocolate mixture over the berries, then pop into the freezer to set for 30 minutes. To serve, either break into shards or cut into wedges.

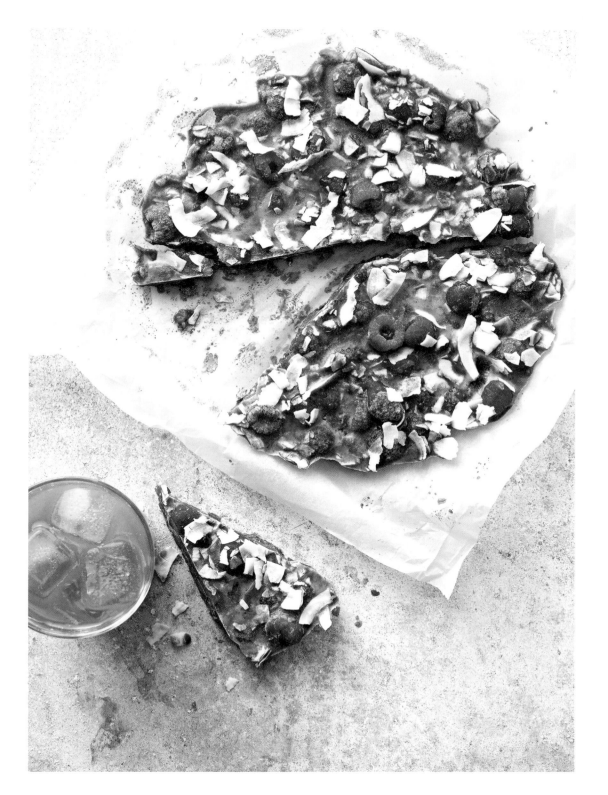

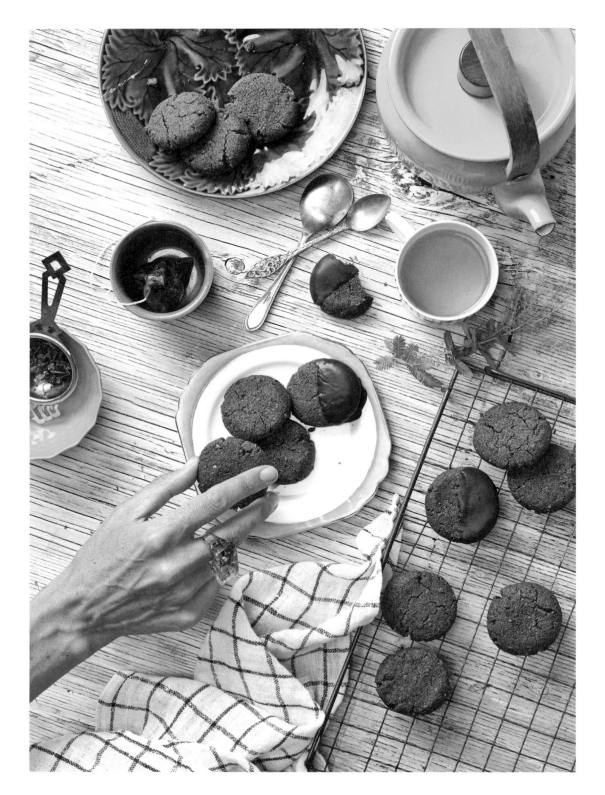

MOCHA CHIP COOKIES

Cookies with chocolate and coffee? Enough said. Once you try one of these cookies, you'll be reaching for another one rather quickly!

SERVES 30

PREPARATION TIME
15 minutes

COOKING TIME
8 minutes

2½ cups (250 g) almond meal

½ teaspoon bicarbonate of soda

½ teaspoon sea salt

120 g butter, softened

1 tablespoon granulated stevia, powdered

1 teaspoon vanilla powder

½ cup (60 g) cacao nibs

3 tablespoons raw cacao powder

1½ tablespoons coffee, ground

1. Preheat the oven to 180°C (gas 4) and line a baking tray with baking paper.
2. Pulse the almond meal, bicarbonate of soda and salt briefly in a food processor. Add the rest of the ingredients and blend a little more. Spoon heaped tablespoons of the mixture onto the baking tray and press down with your hand to flatten.
3. Bake for about 8 minutes until golden. Cool on wire racks before serving.

CHOC-CHIP
SKILLET COOKIE

*This novelty-sized Choc-Chip Cookie is the simplest dessert to bring
along to your next dinner party as it's all made in the one frying pan.
Outrageous!*

SERVES 8

PREPARATION TIME
10 minutes

COOKING TIME
15 minutes

60 g butter

1 tablespoon rice malt syrup

1 teaspoon vanilla extract

1 egg

2 cups (200 g) almond meal

1 teaspoon baking powder

pinch of sea salt

**50 g dark chocolate (85–90%
cocoa), roughly chopped**

thickened cream, to serve

1. Preheat the oven to 180°C (gas 4).

2. Place a small ovenproof frying pan on the stove on low–medium
   heat. Add in butter, rice malt syrup and vanilla and stir until melted
   together. Remove from the heat and allow to cool slightly.

3. Crack egg into the pan and lightly whisk with a fork to combine.
   Add in almond meal, baking powder and salt and stir until a batter
   is formed. Fold through the chocolate pieces.

4. Flatten the mixture around the pan with a spatula. Place in the
   oven and cook for 15 minutes, until very lightly brown on top.

5. Remove from the oven and serve immediately with thickened cream.
   For an optional extra, drizzle with Basic Raw Chocolate (see page 13).

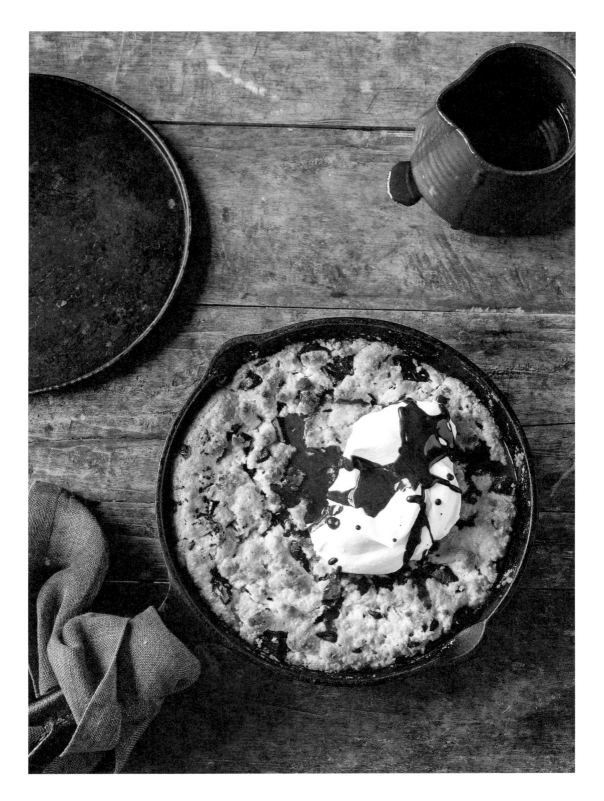

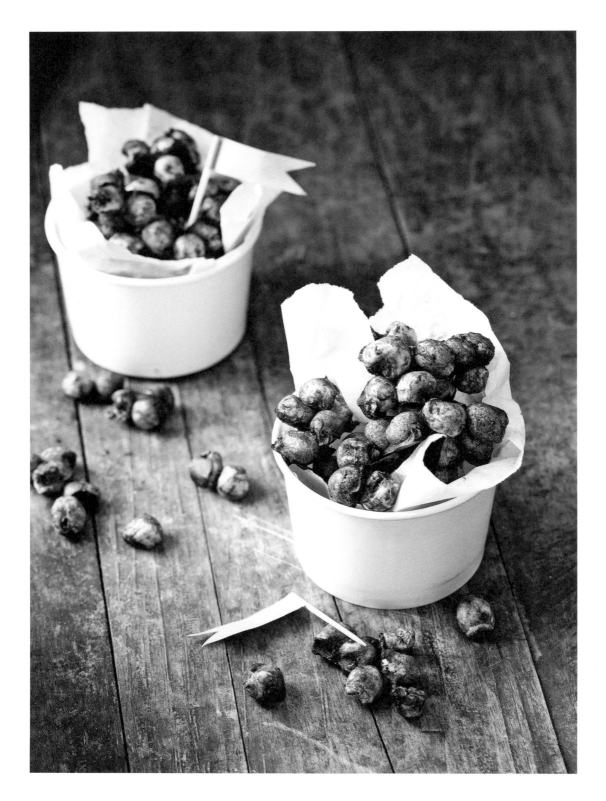

DARK CHOC AND SEA SALT POPCORN

This is a yummy treat to have ready at kids' parties or when mates come over to watch a movie. Warning: you may need to make more!

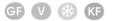

SERVES 2

PREPARATION TIME
30 minutes

COOKING TIME
5 minutes

4 tablespoons coconut oil, melted

2 tablespoons rice malt syrup

3 tablespoons raw cacao powder

pinch of sea salt

1½ cups (40 g) sugar-free puffed rice or corn (or air-popped popcorn)

1. Line a baking tray with baking paper.

2. In a bowl mix coconut oil, rice malt syrup, cacao and salt until smooth. Add puffed rice or corn and stir until coated with mixture.

3. Pour onto lined baking tray and refrigerate for 30 minutes or freeze for 15 minutes before serving.

SUPERFOOD FLORENTINES

Florentines are often super sweet and coated in sugar. We've reworked them to be super healthy treats to fuel you in between meals. If you don't have the exact ingredients throw in any combination of nuts and seeds.

SERVES 8

PREPARATION TIME
30 minutes

COOKING TIME
2 minutes

⅓ cup (40 g) cashews, roughly chopped

⅓ cup (50 g) pistachios, roughly chopped

½ cup (70 g) almonds, roughly chopped

2 tablespoons chia seeds

1–2 tablespoons coconut flakes or desiccated coconut

1 tablespoon rice malt syrup

2 tablespoons coconut oil, melted

40 g dark chocolate (85% cocoa), chopped into even-sized pieces

1. Line a cupcake tin with eight paper cases or baking paper.

2. In a small mixing bowl combine all of the ingredients except for the chocolate.

3. Spoon ingredients into paper cases and flatten with the back of a spoon. Sit Florentines in the freezer to set.

4. Meanwhile, line a plate or tray with baking paper and melt the chocolate over a double boiler or in a microwave until smooth. Dip each Florentine in the chocolate to coat one side. Place on the plate and return to the freezer.

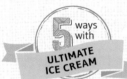

ULTIMATE
ICE CREAM

CHOC-ESPRESSO AND CHILLI ICE CREAM WITH SMASHED ESPRESSO CHOCOLATE

This recipe came about on the day of our photo shoot. We decided to throw together a few of our favourite treats from the day. We were pleasantly surprised by how amazing it tasted. The extra caffeine hit was welcomed, too.

SERVES 6–8

PREPARATION TIME

6 hours

2 tablespoons instant coffee granules

1 teaspoon chilli powder, optional

½ cup (120 ml) Basic Raw Chocolate (see page 13)

1 x 400 ml can coconut cream, chilled

4 pieces of Espresso Truffle (see page 36), roughly chopped

1. Stir coffee and chilli powder with ¼ cup of boiling water until dissolved.

2. Place into a large mixing bowl with Basic Raw Chocolate and coconut cream. Using an electric beater, combine the mixture until it is light and fluffy. The more air you get in this step, the lighter your ice cream will be.

3. Spoon ice cream into a freezer-safe container. Freeze for 6 hours, or until set.

4. Allow ice cream to soften slightly before serving. Serve with chopped-up pieces of Espresso Truffle.

2 SALTED MALT ICE CREAM WITH CARAMEL CRUNCH, CASHEW SWIRLS AND DARK CHOC CHUNKS

If you're a fan of caramel then look no further than this delectable ice cream creation. The crunch of 'activated groaties' throughout makes it even more special.

SERVES 6–8

PREPARATION TIME
6 hours 30 minutes

COOKING TIME
30 seconds

ICE CREAM

1 x 400 ml can coconut cream, chilled

2 tablespoons rice malt syrup

1 teaspoon maca powder

2 teaspoons vanilla powder or extract, optional

pinch of sea salt

2 tablespoons cashew butter

50 g dark chocolate (85% cocoa), chopped into pieces

CARAMEL CRUNCH

2 tablespoons cashew butter

2 tablespoons coconut cream

1 teaspoon rice malt syrup

¾ cup (120 g) 'activated groaties' (activated buckwheat groats)

1. For the Caramel Crunch, add the cashew butter, coconut cream and rice malt syrup to a microwave-proof dish. Microwave for 30 seconds, remove and stir through the activated groaties. Spread onto a baking tray lined with baking paper and place in the freezer to set for 30 minutes.

2. Place all ingredients for the ice cream, except the chocolate, in a large mixing bowl. Using an electric beater, blend the mixture until light and fluffy. The more air you get in this step, the lighter your ice cream will be.

3. Remove the Caramel Crunch from the freezer and break half of it into small pieces. Return remaining half to the freezer. Stir through the ice cream. Add dark chocolate pieces and stir again.

4. Spoon ice cream into a freezer-safe container. Freeze for 6 hours, or until ice cream is set. Allow to soften slightly and sprinkle with broken-up remaining Caramel Crunch before serving.

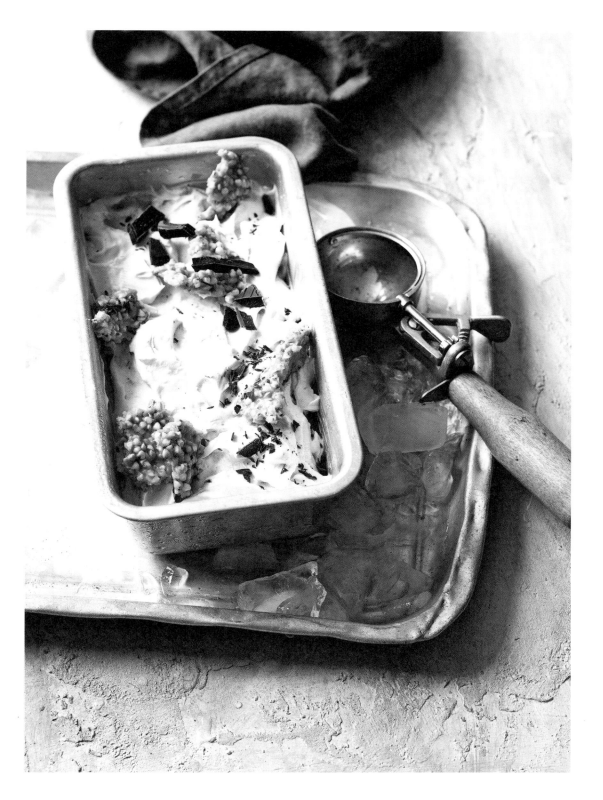

3 VANILLA ICE CREAM WITH A CHOC SWIRL AND VANILLA BUTTERED POPCORN

This one is for vanilla ice cream lovers. The buttered popcorn adds a surprising saltiness to a sweet dessert.

SERVES 6–8

PREPARATION TIME
6 hours

COOKING TIME
5 minutes

ICE CREAM

1 x 400 ml can coconut cream, chilled

2 teaspoons vanilla powder or extract, optional

pinch of sea salt

¼ cup (60 ml) Basic Raw Chocolate (see page 13)

POPCORN

2 cups (25 g) air-popped popcorn

2 tablespoons butter, melted

1 teaspoon vanilla extract

pinch of sea salt

1. For the ice cream, place coconut cream, vanilla and salt in a large mixing bowl. Using an electric beater, blend the mixture until light and fluffy. The more air you get in this step, the lighter your ice cream will be. Place ice cream in a freezer-safe container. Carefully pour in Basic Raw Chocolate and stir through with a spoon to create a swirl.

2. Freeze for 6 hours.

3. Meanwhile, prepare the popcorn by tossing the popcorn, butter, vanilla and salt together in a large bowl. Set aside.

4. Allow ice cream to soften slightly before serving. Serve with popcorn layered throughout.

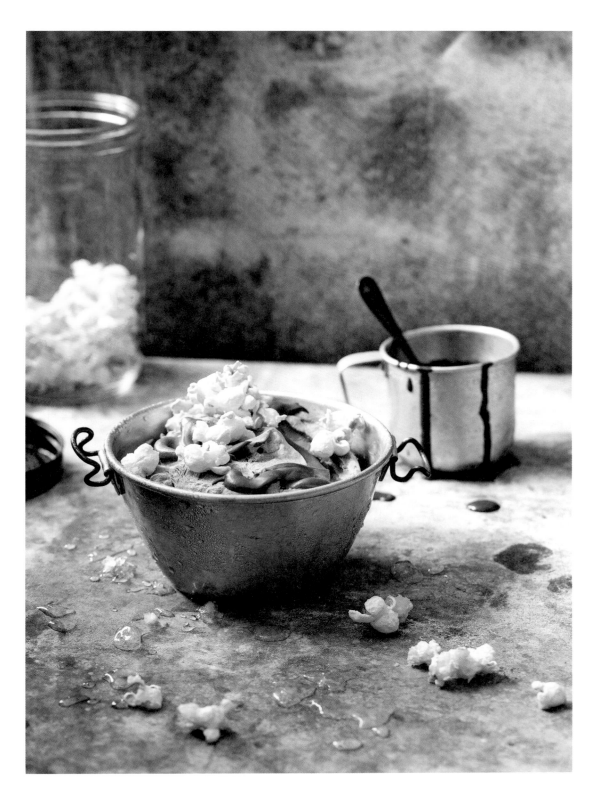

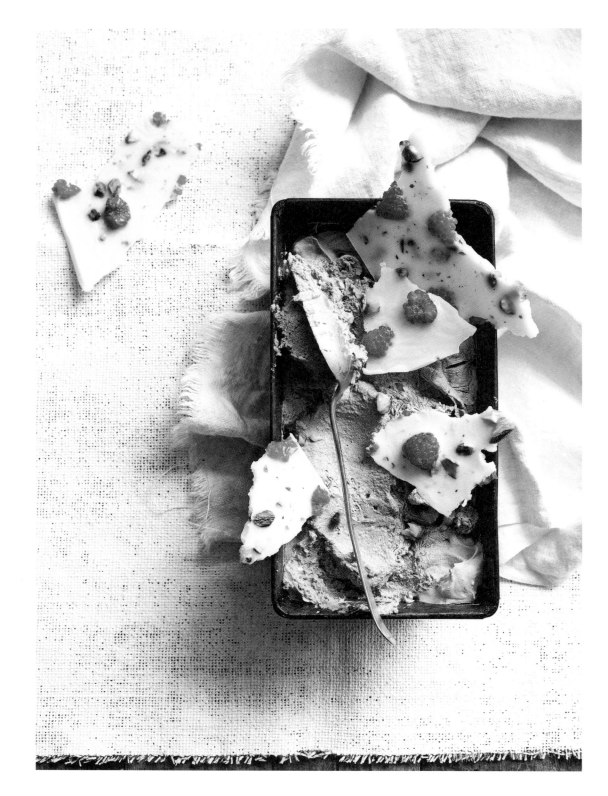

4 DARK CHOCOLATE ICE CREAM WITH WHITE CHOCOLATE, PISTACHIO AND RASPBERRY BARK

This one literally blew our minds. It's like all the tastes of Christmas in one crunchy bite!

SERVES 6–8

PREPARATION TIME
6 hours

1 x 400 ml can coconut cream, chilled

1 cup (250 ml) Basic Raw Chocolate (see page 13)

pinch of sea salt

½ batch of White Christmas Bark (see page 49)

1. Place coconut cream, Basic Raw Chocolate and salt in a large mixing bowl. Using an electric blender, blend the mixture until light and fluffy. The more air you get in this step, the lighter your ice cream will be.

2. Spoon ice cream into a freezer-safe container. Freeze for 6 hours.

3. Allow ice cream to soften slightly before serving. Serve with broken-up pieces of White Christmas Bark.

5 CHOCOLATE ICE CREAM WITH SMASHED CHOCOLATE PEANUT BUTTER 'N' JELLY BROWNIE AND RAW CHOCOLATE SAUCE

Warning: this is super indulgent and should be shared between eight friends, spoons at the ready double-dipping and all.

SERVES 6–8

PREPARATION TIME
6 hours

1 x 400 ml coconut cream, chilled

¼ cup (25 g) raw cacao powder

2 tablespoons rice malt syrup

¼ cup (60 ml) Basic Raw Chocolate (see page 13)

4 pieces of Molten Peanut Butter 'n' Jelly Brownies (see page 108)

1. Place coconut cream, cacao and rice malt syrup in a large mixing bowl. Using an electric beater, blend the mixture until light and fluffy. The more air you get in this step, the lighter your ice cream will be.

2. Spoon ice cream into a freezer-safe container, pour in the Basic Raw Chocolate and create a swirl with a spoon. Place in freezer for 6 hours, or until set.

3. Allow ice cream to soften slightly before serving. Serve with broken-up pieces of Molten Peanut Butter 'n' Jelly Brownies tossed throughout.

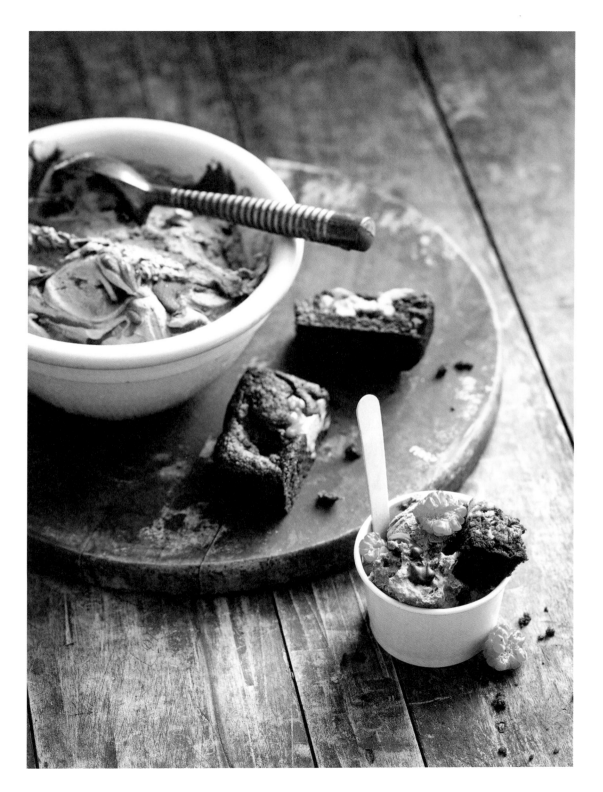

BEETROOT RED VELVET CUPCAKES

If there's an opportunity to make a dessert more nutritionally dense, we'll do it! In this case, we've grated earthy beetroot into these chocolatey cupcakes.

SERVES 12

PREPARATION TIME
10 minutes

COOKING TIME
40 minutes

2 large beetroots, peeled and grated

2 eggs

½ teaspoon vanilla powder

1 teaspoon ground cinnamon

pinch of sea salt

1½ cups (150 g) almond meal

⅓ cup (30 g) raw cacao powder

¼ cup (50 g) coconut oil, melted

⅓ cup (75 ml) rice malt syrup

1 teaspoon baking powder

Cream Cheese Frosting (see page 159), to serve

1. Preheat the oven to 180°C (gas 4) and line a cupcake tin with 12 paper cases.

2. Place all ingredients in a blender and blitz until a smooth batter is formed. Alternatively, you can blend with a stick blender.

3. Divide the mixture between the 12 cases. Bake for 40 minutes.

4. Once cooked through, remove from the oven and allow to cool before topping with Cream Cheese Frosting.

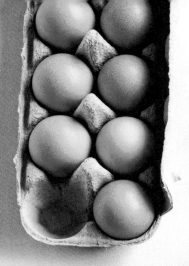

A SUGAR-FREE EASTER

Why not try a sugar-free Easter?
We guarantee these recipes will excite
your tastebuds and the kids will
love them too!

SURVIVING EASTER

When it comes to Easter, there's no shortage of temptation! We've listed our top tips for getting through Easter without falling off the wagon.

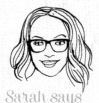

" If you're in an office environment that seems to become festooned with chocolate throughout April, nominate one day in the office where everyone cooks a healthy recipe from this cookbook and celebrates. "

Sarah says

- **Eat a nourishing breakfast.** Start the day off well and eat a breakfast of good fats, protein and greens. This will ensure your blood sugar is stabilised making sweet food less appealing.
- **Get outside and get active.** Exercising, even if it's just a light walk, will help you stave off niggling cravings and distract you from all the sweet temptation.
- **Make your own Easter gifts/treats for yourself.** You don't need to deprive yourself at Easter time. Whip up your favourite chocolate recipe from this book and share it with your loved ones.
- **Shift the focus.** Traditionally Easter was celebrated with fresh seafood. Switch up your menu with some sustainable fish.
- **Share the load.** Don't squirrel away your chocolate! Share it with friends and family. This way there will be less temptation after the event.
- **Indulge in some trickery.** Try wrapping grapes in foil or gifts in pretty paper and hiding them around the house or garden. The kids will love the novelty of 'the treasure hunt', and you can rest assured they won't have a sugar crash in the afternoon.
- **Eat dark chocolate.** If your family insists on buying you treats then ask for dark (85–90% cocoa) chocolate. A little bit of this stuff will keep you satisfied and you won't feel left out of the festivities.

EASTER NEST

This is a great recipe to cook up with the kids. Get them involved and enjoying Easter the healthy way.

MAKES 1

PREPARATION TIME
1 hour

COOKING TIME
5 minutes

1 cup (225 g) macadamias

½ cup (120 ml) rice malt syrup

1 teaspoon vanilla powder
or extract, optional

2 tablespoons raw
cacao powder

¼ cup (25 g) desiccated coconut

3 cups (75 g) low-sugar puffed
rice cereal

1. Process macadamias in a blender or using the chopper attachment of a stick blender for 3 minutes, or until the nuts form a smooth paste.

2. Measure out ½ cup (120 ml) of the macadamia butter and put in a large saucepan.

3. Combine the rice malt syrup, vanilla, cacao and coconut in the saucepan with the macadamia butter and place over low heat.

4. Cook mixture until it melts and is well combined.

5. Place puffed rice in a bowl. Remove nut mixture from the heat and pour over the puffed rice. Allow to cool.

6. Flip the bowl you want for your nest upside down and lay baking paper over it, moulding around the bowl. Cover the bowl with the puffed rice mixture to form a nest. Press mixture down to bond.

7. Refrigerate until hard and carefully peel away from the bowl before filling with Easter chocolate.

EGGSHELL BROWNIES

This recipe is a great show stopper! The novelty of peeling back the eggshells to reveal a chocolate brownie will have the kids busting with excitement. Make this dish at Easter rather than loading the kids up with cheap and nasty store-bought guff.

MAKES 12

PREPARATION TIME
15 minutes

COOKING TIME
25 minutes

12 eggs

1 cup (250 ml) Pumpkin Purée (see page 166)

⅓ cup (75 ml) milk

¼ cup (60 ml) rice malt syrup

¼ cup (50 g) coconut oil, melted

2 teaspoons vanilla powder or extract, optional

⅓ cup (40 g) coconut flour

¼ cup (25 g) raw cacao powder

2 teaspoons baking powder

1. Preheat the oven to 180°C (gas 4).

2. Using the pointy end of a sharp knife, pierce the top of 12 eggshells and peel back enough shell so that the opening is big enough to pipe brownie batter into. Shake contents of 10 of the eggs into a bowl to refrigerate for later, and two into a smaller bowl for use now. Wash the eggshells out thoroughly using warm water.

3. Lay crumpled aluminium foil in a cupcake tin, forming bases to stand the eggs. Place the prepared eggshells in the cupcake tin.

4. In a small saucepan mix together the Pumpkin Purée, milk, rice malt syrup and coconut oil. Place over low heat and stir until the mixture begins to melt. Remove from the heat and set aside to cool slightly. Add the vanilla to the reserved eggs and beat until light and fluffy.

5. In a large bowl mix the flour, cacao and baking powder. Add the pumpkin mixture and beaten eggs then stir to combine. Transfer mixture into a piping bag fitted with a round nozzle. Pipe batter into prepared eggshells to about three-quarters full. Bake for 15–20 minutes or until a skewer comes out clean.

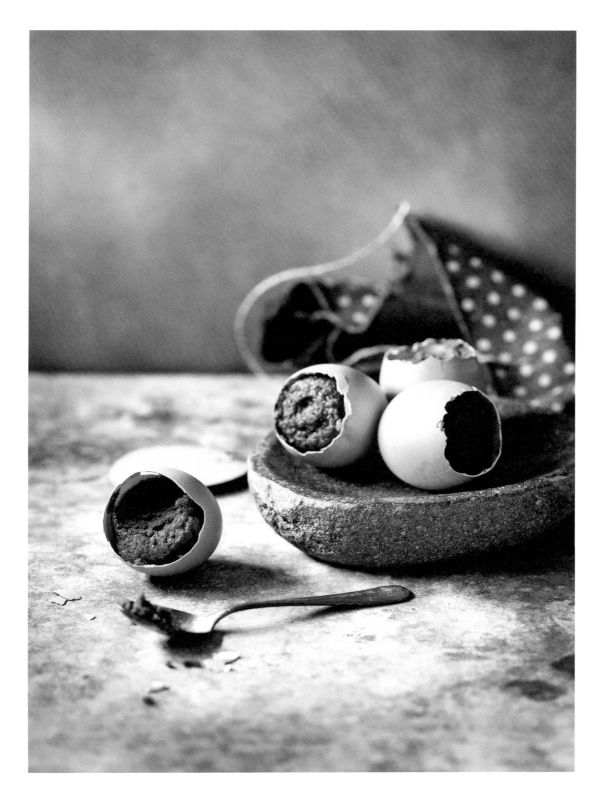

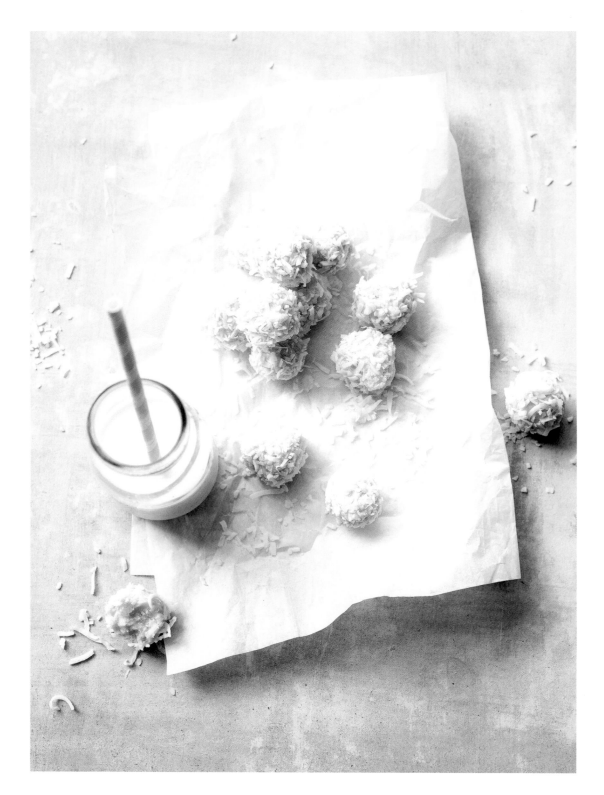

WHITE CHOCOLATE BUNNY TAILS

These are super rich. One serving is all you'll need. But boy, they're good!

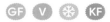

MAKES 20

PREPARATION TIME
1 hour

1¼ cups (300 g) coconut butter

¼ cup (50 g) raw cacao butter, buttons or shavings, melted

¼ cup (50 g) coconut oil

¼ cup (60 ml) coconut milk

¼ cup (60 ml) rice malt syrup

1 teaspoon vanilla powder or extract, optional

pinch of sea salt

shredded coconut, for rolling

1. Place ¼ cup (50 g) coconut butter, cacao butter, coconut oil, coconut milk, rice malt syrup, vanilla and salt in a food processor. Process until smooth.

2. Transfer mixture to a bowl and refrigerate for 20–30 minutes until firmed up enough to roll into balls but not so much that the mixture is solid. Roll mixture into teaspoon-sized balls. Refrigerate until hard.

3. Mould remaining coconut butter in a thin layer around each ball and then roll in shredded coconut. Refrigerate until firm.

CHOCOLATE PEANUT BUTTER HOT COCOA

The perfect match – peanut butter and chocolate. This warming drink recipe is the perfect pick-me-up treat for a cool afternoon.

SERVES 2

PREPARATION TIME
10 minutes

1 x 400 ml can coconut milk

½ cup (120 ml) almond milk

1 teaspoon rice malt syrup, or to taste

2 tablespoons natural, sugar-free peanut butter

½ cup (50 g) raw cacao powder

pinch of sea salt, to taste

2 tablespoons cacao nibs

1. Throw all ingredients except the cacao nibs into a saucepan and whisk like crazy. Bring to a low boil, then simmer for several minutes while whisking to remove any remaining clumps. Pour mixture into two mugs and top with cacao nibs to serve.

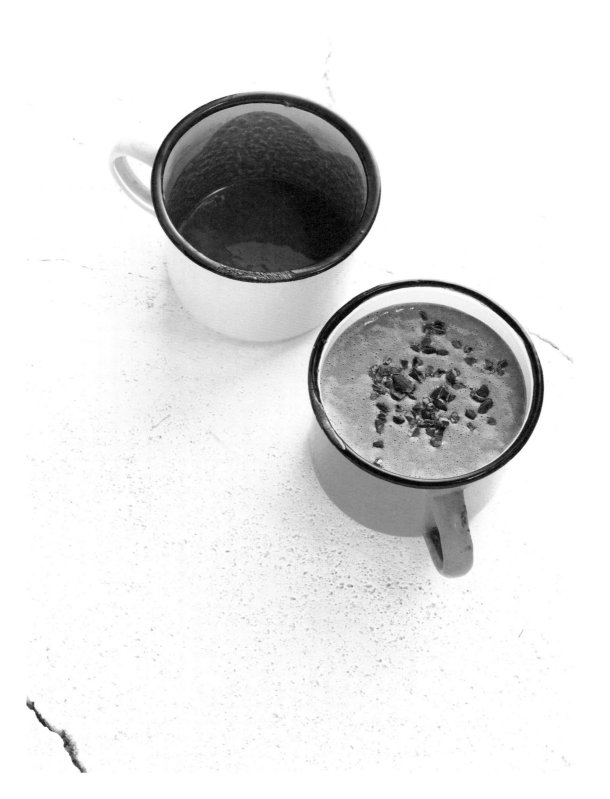

CHOC-CHIP HOT CROSS BUNS

Did you know you can rise yeast without sugar? Which means you can make your favourite traditional recipes, only healthier, like these Choc-Chip Hot Cross Buns. Serve with a generous slather of butter.

SERVES 15

PREPARATION TIME
1 hour 35 minutes

COOKING TIME
20 minutes

1 tablespoon dried yeast

4¾ cups (475 g) spelt flour

1½ cups (375 ml) full-fat milk, lukewarm (not hot otherwise it will kill the yeast)

1 teaspoon rice malt syrup

1 teaspoon sea salt

1 tablespoon granulated stevia

1 teaspoon ground cinnamon

½ teaspoon allspice

60 g butter, at room temperature

1 egg, lightly beaten

50 g dark chocolate (85–90% cocoa), chopped finely

GLAZE

2 teaspoons rice malt syrup

1 tablespoon boiling water

1. Mix yeast, 1 tablespoon spelt flour, warm milk and rice malt syrup in a mixing bowl. Cover and stand in a warm place for 15 minutes until mixture is frothy.

2. Meanwhile, sift 4 cups (400 g) of the spelt flour, salt, stevia and spices into a large bowl and toss to combine. Add in the butter and rub with your fingers until combined.

3. Once the yeast mixture is frothy, add to the flour mix with the whisked egg. Stir to combine. Add in the chocolate pieces then fold through. Cover the bowl again and allow to stand in a warm place for 40 minutes or until dough has almost doubled in size.

4. Preheat the oven to 200°C (gas 6) and lightly grease an 18 cm x 30 cm baking tin.

5. Punch dough down, turn onto a floured surface, and knead well until dough is smooth and elastic. Cut into three equal pieces then cut each piece into five. Knead each into a round shape.

6. Place buns in the prepared tin in rows. Don't worry if they don't touch, they will expand in the oven. Cover and allow to stand for 10–15 minutes in a warm place or until the buns have expanded.

7. Meanwhile, to make the crosses, sift remaining spelt flour into a bowl and add ¼ cup (60 ml) of water, mix to form a paste. You may need to add a touch more water to make the mixture a thick, but still fluid, consistency. Place in a small ziplock bag and then cut a hole across the corner. Use this to pipe crosses onto the top of each bun.

8. Place buns in the oven and bake for 20 minutes.

9. Meanwhile, combine the rice malt syrup with boiling water. Once hot cross buns have cooked, remove from the oven and immediately brush with glaze. Serve buns warm with a generous slather of butter.

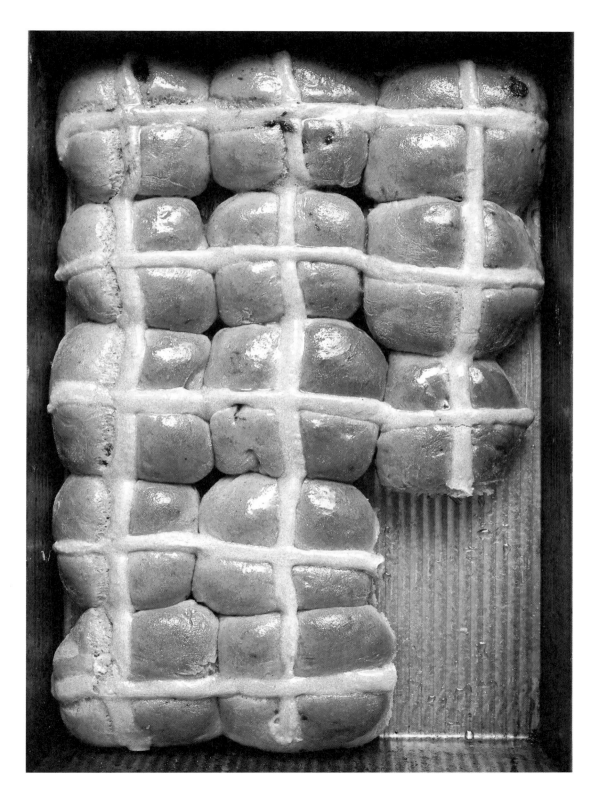

WHITE CHOCOLATE RASPBERRY RIPPLE EASTER BUNNIES

Trick the kids into thinking they're eating real white chocolate with these yummy treats.

GF V ❄ KF

MAKES 6

PREPARATION TIME
30 minutes

COOKING TIME
5 minutes

½ cup (115 g) raw cacao butter, buttons or shavings

½ cup (100 g) coconut oil

1 teaspoon vanilla powder or extract, optional

pinch of sea salt

1 tablespoon rice malt syrup

½ cup (60 g) frozen raspberries, defrosted

1. Add cacao butter, coconut oil, vanilla, sea salt and rice malt syrup to a small pan over low temperature. Whisk until everything has melted and combined.

    Note: The rice malt syrup will drop to the bottom of the pan. Ensure you whisk really well to combine the syrup into the chocolate.

2. Add chopped raspberries to a bunny or other Easter-themed mould. Pour over white chocolate and place in the freezer for at least 30 minutes to set before serving.

TWELVE BASIC FROSTINGS, SAUCES AND BUTTERS

*Refer back to this chapter whenever
you're after the perfect frosting for a cake
or the best sauce for your pancakes.*

COCONUT BUTTER

*You can buy this stuff in health food shops, but it can be expensive.
Or you can make your own cheaply and in minutes for a surprisingly
white chocolate-like hit.*

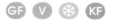

MAKES ¾ cup
(175 ml)

PREPARATION TIME
15 minutes

**1 packet (250 g) shredded coconut
(bigger is better; you can also use
coconut flakes or desiccated coconut)**

1. Using a high-powered food processor, process for about 3 minutes
   (a regular blender will take up to 15 minutes and requires a lot of
   scraping and stirring) until a runny butter forms.

2. Scrape the sides of the bowl as necessary. Store in a jar either at room
   temperature or in the fridge, depending on the season and climate.

TRICKY TIP
- - - - - - - - - -

Use coconut butter as a soft spreadable paste on toast, sprinkled with
salt. If you store the coconut butter in the fridge, you'll need to 'cut out'
a chunk and soften it at room temperature before using.

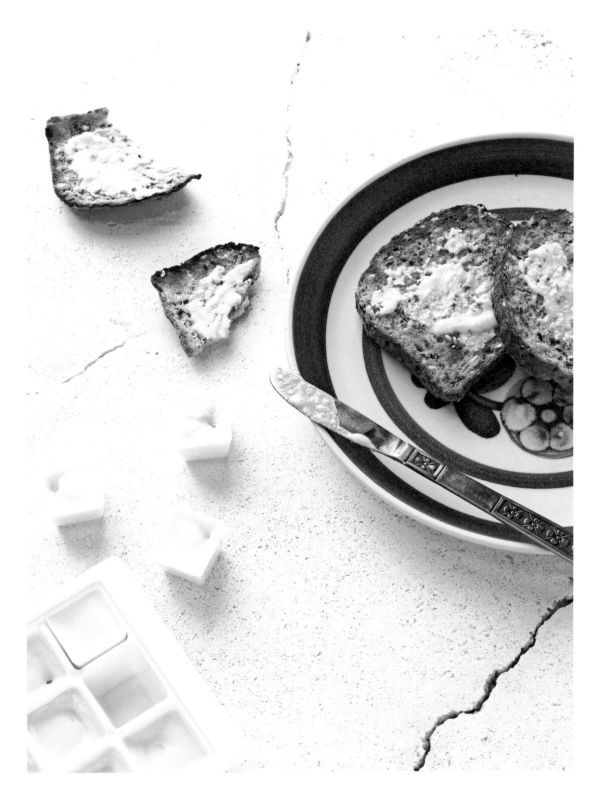

CHOCOLATE COCONUT BUTTER

You might want to make this in bulk and store it in ice cube trays so you can pull out one or two for toast, pancakes or a smoothie, or for a little ganachey treat with your tea in the afternoon.

MAKES ⅓ cup
(75 ml)

PREPARATION TIME
15 minutes

3 tablespoons Coconut Butter (see page 156), softened or melted

1½ teaspoons raw cacao powder

2 tablespoons hazelnut meal, optional

1. Using a teaspoon, mix all the ingredients in a small cup until blended (the cacao powder requires a bit of 'smashing' to ensure all the lumps disappear).

2. Refrigerate or freeze until firm.

WHIPPED COCONUT CREAM

This cream is great with a brownie or cupcake (in lieu of ice cream or cream). You can also use it as a frosting.

MAKES 1 cup
(250 ml)

PREPARATION TIME
freeze overnight

1 x 400 ml can full-fat coconut cream

1 tablespoon granulated stevia

1. Place can upside down in the fridge overnight (be sure not to shake the can beforehand). The next day, turn the can right way up and open without shaking it. Spoon out the top layer of liquid (and keep for smoothies or other recipes requiring coconut milk or coconut water).

2. Leave the rest of the harder cream in the can, add stevia and then blend with a stick blender until creamy. (If you don't have a stick blender, remove the cream from the can and blend with beaters or in a blender.)

CREAM CHEESE FROSTING

This works best in recipes that aren't too sweet. Try it with the Chocolate Red Velvet Cake (see page 95).

MAKES 1 cup
(250 ml)

PREPARATION TIME
5 minutes

250 g cream cheese

½ lemon, juice and zest, optional

2 teaspoons rice malt syrup

3 tablespoons coconut cream

1. Blend cheese in a high-speed blender along with the lemon juice and zest, if using, and the rice malt syrup.

2. Slowly add the coconut cream until the mixture is nice and thick. If needed, add more coconut cream until it's thick enough.

CHOCOLATE BUTTERCREAM FROSTING

This frosting tastes great on any cupcake.

MAKES 1 cup
(250 ml)

PREPARATION TIME
5 minutes

⅓ cup (75 g) unsalted butter, at room temperature

2 tablespoons rice malt syrup

⅓ cup (30 g) raw cocoa powder

1 teaspoon vanilla powder or extract, optional

1. In a mixing bowl combine all ingredients and whisk until thoroughly combined and fluffy.

> **TRICKY TIP**
>
> For a firmer frosting, set mixture in the fridge for 15 minutes.

CHOCOLATE MOUSSE FROSTING

This stuff can be eaten on its own, or as a dip with strawberries for dessert.

MAKES 1 cup
(250 ml)

PREPARATION TIME
5 minutes

1½ tablespoons rice malt syrup

2 ripe avocados

1 teaspoon vanilla extract or paste

¼ cup (25 g) raw cacao powder

2 tablespoons coconut milk
(or milk of your choice) or water

1. Blend all ingredients but the milk in a high-speed blender until creamy and thick (a stick blender can also work).

2. Add a tablespoon or two of milk or water to achieve a smooth texture.

CASHEW FROSTING

This stuff is lush. Use it as a spread on a brownie or even a slice of toast.

MAKES 1 cup
(250 ml)

PREPARATION TIME
5 minutes

1 cup (135 g) raw cashews, soaked in water overnight, drained

1½ tablespoons rice malt syrup

½ lemon, juice and zest

¼ cup (60 ml) coconut cream

1. Blend cashews in a high-speed blender along with the rice malt syrup, lemon juice and zest.

2. Slowly add the coconut cream until the mixture is nice and thick. If needed add more coconut cream until it's thick enough.

ICE MAGIC

*Just like the crazy stuff you had on ice cream as a kid
(with the same crack to the spoon)!*

MAKES 1 cup
(250 ml)

PREPARATION TIME
5 minutes

½ cup (100 g) coconut oil

½ cup (50 g) raw cacao powder

½ tablespoon granulated stevia

pinch of sea salt

1. Melt coconut oil in a small saucepan over low heat and add the rest of
   the ingredients, whisking well to dissolve the stevia.

2. Let cool slightly, and then pour over homemade sugar-free ice cream.

> **TRICKY TIP**
>
> Store in covered container in the refrigerator and melt when you need
> to use it.

PRE-SOAKED CASHEWS

*Soaking cashews helps to eliminate the phytic acid stored in the husk
of nuts, making it easier for the body to digest. Soaking also helps to
make nuts blend more easily.*

MAKES 2 cups
(275 g)

PREPARATION TIME
4 hours

2 cups (275 g) raw cashews

2½ cups (600 ml) water

1. Add cashews and water to a bowl for 2–4 hours. Drain excess water
   and store in the fridge for up to 3 days until needed.

GOOEY CARAMEL SAUCE

It's gooey and caramelly. That's all you need to know.

MAKES 1 cup
(250 ml)

PREPARATION TIME
5 minutes (+ optional cooling time)

COOKING TIME
15 minutes

⅓ cup (75 ml) rice malt syrup

100 g butter, chopped

½ cup (120 ml) coconut cream

1. Heat the rice malt syrup in a pan until bubbling vigorously. If you have a sugar thermometer, heat until the caramel reaches 135°C. If you don't have a thermometer, cook the syrup for 13 minutes until it has reduced down. The mixture should be thick, drippy and lightly coat the back of a spoon.

2. Add butter and stir until combined over medium heat. Remove from heat and slowly add coconut cream, stirring until combined. Pour caramel into a bowl and sit in the freezer for a few hours until thick. Alternatively, pour straight onto a pudding or cake.

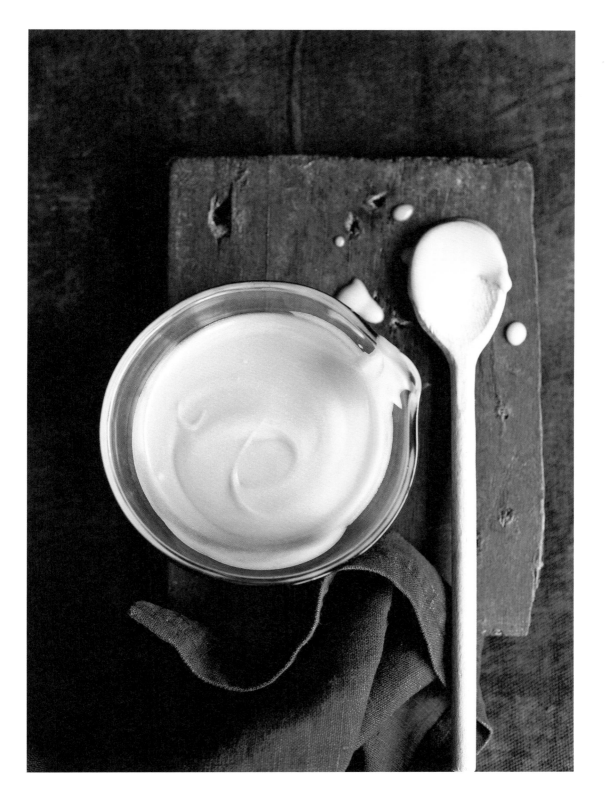

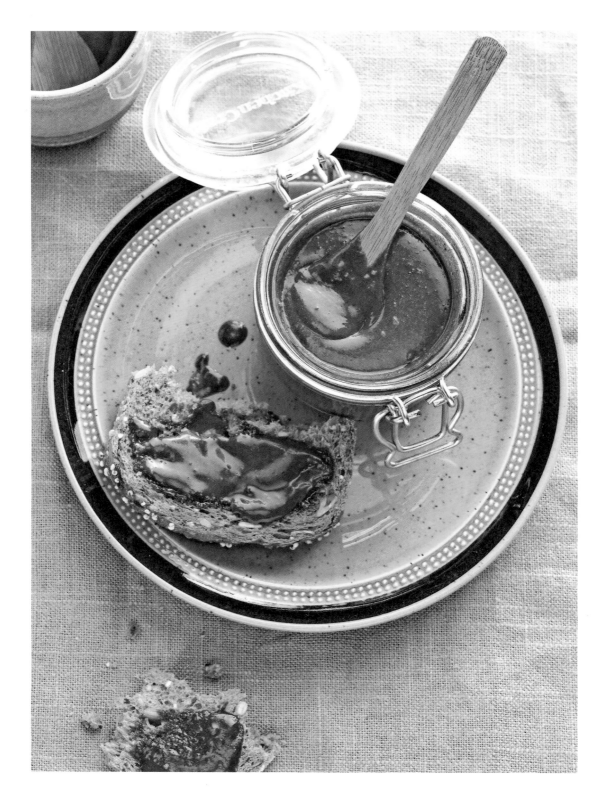

CHOC HAZELNUT SPREAD

Once you taste this version you'll never buy the stuff off the shelves again.

MAKES 1 cup
(250 ml)

PREPARATION TIME
10 minutes

COOKING TIME
10 minutes

1 cup (120 g) hazelnuts

½ cup (120 ml) coconut milk

1 tablespoon rice malt syrup

1 tablespoon coconut oil

¼ cup (25 g) raw cacao powder

2 teaspoons vanilla powder
or extract, optional

1. Preheat the oven to 180°C (gas 4). Bake the hazelnuts on a tray for 8–10 minutes, until browned. Rub off most of the skins as they can be bitter (you don't have to be too precise).

2. Pulse the nuts in a food processor until smooth. Add the remaining ingredients and process until well mixed.

3. Add extra coconut milk if you want more of a 'sauce' consistency.

TRICKY TIP

Store the spread in the fridge for several weeks.

PUMPKIN PURÉE

This is a staple in the IQS kitchen. We use it for cakes, brownies and savoury dishes.

MAKES 2–4 cups
(500 ml–1 litre)

PREPARATION TIME
5 minutes

COOKING TIME
35 minutes

1 large pumpkin (any variety will do), peeled and roughly chopped

5 tablespoons olive oil

1. Preheat the oven to 200°C (gas 6) . Line a baking tray with baking paper.

2. Rub the pumpkin with olive oil, and bake in the oven until tender – about 30–35 minutes.

3. Add pumpkin to a food processor and blitz until smooth. Allow to cool then store separately in one-cup (250 ml) batches in the freezer (in ziplock bags or containers).

SWEET POTATO PURÉE

Just like Pumpkin Purée, sweet potatoes can be cooked and blitzed into a sweet purée to be used as a nutrient-booster in chocolatey desserts.

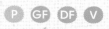

MAKES 3 cups
(750 ml)

PREPARATION TIME
5 minutes

COOKING TIME
35 minutes

1 kg sweet potatoes, left whole and unpeeled

2 tablespoons extra virgin olive oil

pinch of sea salt

1. Preheat the oven to 220°C (gas 7).

2. Rub the sweet potato with olive oil and prick with a fork. Place on a tray in the oven and bake until the skin starts to expand, crisp up and feels soft – about 35 minutes.

3. Once cooked, remove from the oven, cool a little and peel the skin off. Place the sweet potato flesh and the sea salt into a blender and blitz until smooth. Or mash well with a fork.

4. Separate purée into one-cup (250 ml) batches and place into ziplock bags or containers and freeze until needed.

INDEX

CONTRIBUTORS

We got some contributor love on this project, too.

In addition to our recipes, this book features some amazing recipes from our foodie friends. Many thanks to:

Alice Nicholls from The Whole Daily.

Marisa Alvarsson from MissMarzipan.com.

Zainab from Lagallete.com.

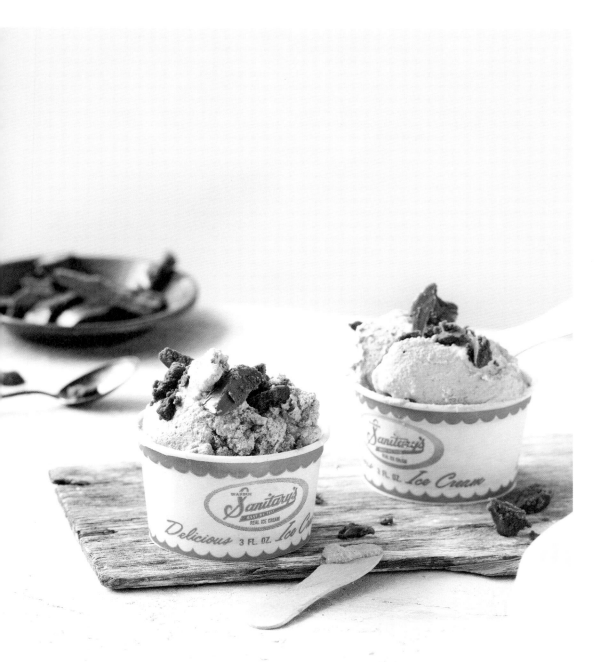

CHOC-ESPRESSO AND CHILLI ICE CREAM WITH SMASHED ESPRESSO CHOCOLATE

THANK YOU

The *I Quit Sugar The Ultimate Chocolate Cookbook* was put together by the I Quit Sugar Team. Thanks to the Pan Macmillan team and the fantastic food photography that was carried out by Jeremy Simons, Michelle Noerianto and Theressa Klein.

Special mention goes out to our contributors and readers who kindly shared their favourite recipes.

First published 2017 by Pan Macmillan Australia Pty Ltd.

First published in the UK 2017 by Bluebird
an imprint of Pan Macmillan
20 New Wharf Road, London N1 9RR
Associated companies throughout the world
www.panmacmillan.com

ISBN 978-1-5098-5836-1

A CIP catalogue record for this book is available from the British Library.

Design by Elissa Webb, adapted from design by Lisa Valuyskaya
Food styling and props by Michelle Noerianto
Food preparation by Theressa Klein

Printed and bound in Italy

Visit **www.panmacmillan.com** to read more about all our books
and to buy them. You will also find features, author interviews and
news of any author events, and you can sign up for e-newsletters
so that you're always first to hear about our new releases.